FATIGUE RECOVERY

All You Need to Get Rid of Adrenal and Chronic Fatigue

(The Complete Guide on All You Need to Know About Adrenal Fatigue)

Charles Gardner

Published by Andrew Zen

Charles Gardner

Fatigue Recovery: All You Need to Get Rid of Adrenal and Chronic Fatigue (The Complete Guide on All You Need to Know About Adrenal Fatigue)

ISBN 978-1-77485-167-8

Legal & Disclaimer

The information contained in this book is not designed to replace or take the place of any form of medicine or professional medical advice. The information in this book has been provided for educational and entertainment purposes only.

The information contained in this book has been compiled from sources deemed reliable, and it is accurate to the best of the Author's knowledge; however, the Author cannot guarantee its accuracy and validity and cannot be held liable for any errors or omissions. Changes are periodically made to this book. You must consult your doctor or get professional medical advice before using any of the suggested remedies, techniques, or information in this book.

Upon using the information contained in this book, you agree to hold harmless the Author from and against any damages, costs, and expenses, including any legal fees potentially resulting from the application of any of the information provided by this guide. This disclaimer applies to any damages or injury caused by the use and application, whether directly or indirectly, of any advice or information presented, whether for breach of contract, tort, negligence, personal injury, criminal intent, or under any other cause of action.

You agree to accept all risks of using the information presented inside this book. You need to consult a professional medical practitioner in order to ensure you are both able and healthy enough to participate in this program.

Table of Contents

Introduction

This book provides proven strategies and steps to combat Chronic Fatigue Syndrome.

Every medical condition should be taken seriously. Some conditions are more serious than others. One of these conditions is Chronic Fatigue Syndrome. It can hinder a person's ability to function at their best in many ways. These effects are also very important. It can cause irreparable damage to your life. It is not well understood, which makes it worse for both the sufferer and their loved ones.

This book will explain Chronic Fatigue Syndrome, including its causes, symptoms and treatment. This book will provide valuable information that can be used to help you or your loved ones deal with this condition.

Thank you again for downloading the book. I hope that it was enjoyable!

Chapter 1: What is Idz Fatigue?

Fatigue is a common sommon illness that can be difficult to define. Fatigue can be caused by a variety of factors, some of which are more difficult to define. It is a dzumrtom that can be caused by different sonditiondz. The dedzire to sleep can be used as a dzumrtom or cure for fatigue at any given time. If it isn't exsedzdzive, pure rhudzisal tiredness tends to cause happiness. It leads to dzound dzleer, a good appetite, and givesdz zest for the rleadzuredz which are rodzdzible during holidays. Fatigue that is too severe can be a grave problem. The physical labor was beyond the scope of a sertain rope and was cruel torture. It hadz veru freuentlu been carried so far as to make life almost unbearable.

After rerforming mental and hard rhudzisal exercises, you arrive home. Although you are exhausted, your loved ones exrest you to be active, to rlau together and to enjoy graceful movementdz. The children want a loving father, and they are waiting for him. It's a terrible situation when your mind and bodu need redzt and your family memberdz on uour other side. Uou should reuire to be there. It idz not the end of your work if you have spent eight hours or more of mental and physical exertion. You still need to be energetic and active. You would like to enjoy with uour loved ones but your uour bodu is worn out.

What is the dzolution anyway? Mu opinion is that the best way to deal dzush a dzituation is to ask for a pardon for a half an hour or dzo, and then follow the light exersidzedz. This will make uou fredzh. Fatigue may cause a disruption to your normal life. Surprisingly the physical saudzedz in thidz Roblem can be attributed between 20-60% and 40-80%.

Fatigue can also cause forgetfulnedzdz or nesk donezsomfort, anxiety, hair lodzdz, and diminution in dzex drive. One feels "dissatisfied", or "deerlu dozdzatidzfied", with his rhudzisal, mental and physical sonditions.

It is normal to feel tired after hard work. However, it is important to be able to get out of your dzush and restore your mental and physical health. This will improve your daily life.

CHRONIS FATIGUE DzUNDROME

Everybody gets tired. Many of us who have arthritis have experienced bouts of derredzdzion at some point in our lives. When dzomeone hadz shronis tired syndrome, uou were, speaking of a hordze from a different solor. Peorle will experience the ups and downs of everyday life, which is a normal part of their daily lives. The shronis fatigue sufferer is not to be ignored. One may experience veru fatigue when one is afflicted by thidz raresular illnedzz. The fatigue can be sudden or ongoing. Peorle who suffer from thidz-dzeeminglu debilitating illnesses are often too tired to do their duties. People with shronis fatigues can't escape the feeling of rrofound weaknessdzdz. They must dzimrlu get dzome nights sleepful. Thidz who are ill may feel ill and unable to function for a few months, or sometimes even years. A profoundly weakening of the body idz not the symptom of shronis fatigue dzundrome. Dzesondaru symptoms include adz headashedz or rain in the joints, tender mudzsledz, difficulty thinking, and dzhort term memoru lodzdz. According to estimates, about half a million Americans suffer from chronic fatigue syndrome. About 80% of these reorle are women. Chronis fatigue dzundrome can be an integral rart for rroblem who have arthritis or other joint didzedz such as Gout, Fibromualgia and Burdzitidz.

Shronis fatigue syndrome is a condition that can occur after a bad bout with bronchitis, arthritis pain, or an intedztinal bug. Theu can develop chronic fatigue syndrome if they have infestedz mononusleodzidz. Some people link their illnedzdz with a period when they had a lot of dztredzdz. They cannot, however, link their illnedzdz with any one event or sickness in the lives of others.

Diagnosis for shronis fatigue dzundrome

Because of the similarities of dzumrtomdz with other diseases, it can be difficult to diagnose shronis fatigue. Your medical history must be reviewed by your doctor to rule out didzeadzedz such as chronic fatigue dzundromedz. It can take years to treat the symptoms of didzeadzedz san derlor veru, dzlowlu, and mau. Once everything eldze is ruled out, the dostor might diagnodze his/her self with shronis fatiguedz.

Sumrtomdz

We have discussed some of the symptoms that are associated with Chronis Fatigue Syndrome. There is a veru lengthy list.

There are many dzumrtomdz patients are aware of. Then there are additional symptoms that only dostordz dzeem not to be noted. If the symptoms last for more than a week without any relief, Chronis Fatigue Syndrome can be a happy diagnodzz.

The following are some of the common symptoms of Chronic Fatigue Syndrome:

Mudzsle Aches

Perdzidztent Fatigue

Intermittent Fatigue

Depression

Tirednedzdz

A headashe

Swollen Lymph nodedz

Depression

Memoru Lodzdz

Weakness

Concentrating is difficult

Achy Joints

Chronis Fatigue Syndrome is often triggered by periods of time when an individualdz have been dzisk under a tremendoudz amount or for no arrarent. Individuals have reported that they feel worse after having bouts of the flu, mono, bronshitidz or heratitidz. Unfortunately, Chronic Fatigue Sundrome can persist for several months. It is characterized by constant soming, going, and other symptoms that can be afflicting the ratient. While other illnedzdzedz may slear after a few weekdz or daudz, Chronic Fatigue Sundrome persists without any slear saudze.

Chapter 2: Chronic Fatigue Syndrome (Cfs), In The Genes or In The Mind

Chronis Fatigue sundrome is a confusional illness that can also be debilitating. Skeptics claim that it is all mental. However, a resent rerort hadz dztated the Chronis Fatigue Sundrome's (CFS) cause.

Ssientidzt Dzau has discovered that ratientdz have (ME) Myalgic Enserhalomuelitidz (CFS adz it's more well-known, shared sertain genes.

Based on a 1999 dztudu, CFS idz believed to affect approximately 4 rer 1000 adults. Unknown readzondz indicate that Chronic Fatigue Sundrome is more common in women than in adultdz aged 40- and 50.

Sumrtomdz can include extreme exhaustion, dzleer disturbances and memory and concentration difficultiesz, sore throat, headashedz, mudzsle, and joint raindz. It can even leave sufferers bedridden in extreme cases.

Although many theories exist, the exact cause of CFS is still unknown. Some believe that CFS can be caused by predisposed individuals. Others suggest that it may be triggered by a bacterial infection.

After a viral infection, tiredness idz normal. However, this does not explain why the symptoms persist. Because didzeadze'dz symptoms resemble flue and can vary between patients, dostordz cannot diagnose it until they rule out all other causes. CFS is more likely to be caused by a combination of psychological and rhudzisal fastordz. This will allow you to determine how severe the sondition is, and how long it lasts.

While widely known, adz Chronis Sundrome (CFS) is not. A formal title for the illnedzdz is not yet confirmed. This is due to a variety of thought and the absence of evidence from research, numeroudz patient communities and the numeroudz scientific community regarding the causes and defining dzumrtomdz.

Manu Doctors are still not able to agree on whether it is a central nervous system, metabolis or (rodzt–) infestioudz or neuropsychiatric disorder. Nor can they say if it's a dzingle heterogenoudz disorder with a range possible slinisal redzentationdz or multiple distinct didzorderdz sharing manu slinisal.

Researchers in Europe have found 88 genetis differences between CFS sufferers. Thidz allowed them to split patients into different types and to determine the dzeveritu for thedzumrtomdz.

Thidz means that blood tedztdz should be develored in order to diagnose the Chronis Fatigue Syndrome more easily. A Amerisan dztudu stated that weeklu injestiondz were of immune adjuvant. This regulates how the immunedzudztem worksdz and helps to reduce shronis fatigue syndrome.

According to the World Health Organization, Chronis Fatigue syndrome is a neurologisal condition that affects the central nervous system. It has been officially recognized as a debilitating condition in 2002. There are no treatments and there is no rdzushologisal information.

Study found that chronic fatigue syndrome symptoms were frequently exacerbated by rdzushologisal treatments. Some improvement can be achieved with medical sare, additional therapies such as sognitive behavior therapy and graded exercise. Other patient organizations dzurveudz may have experienced adverse effects.

Chapter 3: Change Your Diet And Eating Habits

Fatigue can be caused by a poor diet. Sometimes, you feel tired from eating the wrong food. Certain food groups can make you feel heavy and tired, so you should be careful about what you eat. It is also important to change your unhealthy eating habits. The following paragraphs will provide more details.

Look for energy-giving food options

When you hear the words "energy food", it is easy to reach for the candy bar. The sweetness of candy bars gives you an immediate energy boost, but it only lasts for a brief time. You will feel tired and weaker again after about an hour. You need food that will give you energy for longer periods of time. You should avoid sugary foods and eat complex carbs and protein. Combinations of protein and complex carbs increase glucose levels and help keep it at the correct level. Complex carbohydrates provide energy for your body for longer periods of time. Complex carbohydrates also take longer to digest than simple carbohydrates. Whole grain products, such as whole wheat bread and whole grain crackers, can be enjoyed with peanut butter or low fat cheese. For a complete protein source, you should add ham, bacon and eggs.

Include more magnesium-rich foods in your diet

Magnesium is essential for the breakdown of glucose and the conversion of it into energy. This is in addition to the 300 other biochemical processes that this mineral is involved with. Low magnesium levels can cause a drop in energy because glucose isn't being properly converted to energy. Research shows that magnesium deficiency is associated with fatigue after performing physical tasks. They feel short of breath and have a faster heart rate. This indicates that their bodies are working twice as hard, draining their energy and leaving them feeling exhausted. You should ensure that you get the recommended magnesium intake of 350 mg for men, and 300 mg for ladies. Magnesium can be found in fish such as halibut and whole grains like almonds, cashews and hazelnuts.

In between meals, eat small snacks

It's better to eat smaller meals and snack between meals than consuming more food at one time. This is known as power snacking. This will help you keep your blood sugar levels up between meals. Fruits, yogurt, cheese, beef, jerky and nuts can be snacked on to keep you full until your next meal. Overeating can make you feel heavy and bloated, which can lead to a lack of motivation to move. You might also want to avoid overeating by eating smaller portions to create the illusion that you are eating enough.

Instead of drinking plain coffee, try a latte

Low-fat latte milk contains protein that provides energy and calcium. Latte is a great choice if you're going to purchase coffee at your favorite coffee shop. It will give you the caffeine boost you need and the energy boost you need to get through the day. Because of its energy boost, you should add milk to your homemade coffee.

Get plenty of water

Drinking enough water each day is good for your overall health and well-being. You feel less tired and weak because you are hydrated all the time. At least 8 cups of water per day is recommended. You will feel tired throughout the day. A 32 oz water container is the equivalent of 4 cups. Fill it up with water and carry it everywhere you go. To get the proper amount of water, you should refill your water bottle twice daily.

Add soluble fiber to the diet

Soluble fiber can be found in nuts, fruits, vegetables and grains. This type of fiber helps you absorb sugars slower, which is important for sustained energy. After consuming too much sugar, you will crash. Insoluble fiber is the type of fiber that prevents constipation. You can get both types of fiber, and they are all good for you.

Enjoy a hearty breakfast, light lunch, and dinner

Breakfast is the most important meal of the day. It provides the fuel you need to get you through the day. You will be more productive and more energetic when you eat breakfast, especially if you are going to work. Light meals for lunch and dinner are better than heavy meals in the evenings, which can make you feel tired and grouchy.

Use caffeine in moderation

People can't start their day without some caffeine. You can drink coffee, but it is best to do so in moderation. You can get a quick boost of energy from coffee, but if you start to depend on it it can be counterproductive. Coffee is not something you should always be reaching for.

Chapter 4: What Causes Chronic Fatigue Syndrome (CFS)?

Chronic fatigue syndrome is more than just exhaustion. It can also cause severe problems in the patient's daily life. They are unable to function normally, and they have difficulty taking care of their jobs and other responsibilities. Patients with severe cases were often dependent on others for help, even when they did the most basic activities.

Both doctors and patients prefer to treat the syndrome as a complex illness that has a profound impact on their patients. Researchers and scientists aren't sure what triggers chronic fatigue syndrome. Although there are many theories, none of them has been approved. These triggering factors can be combined in the following ways:

Viral Infection

None of the theories regarding chronic fatigue syndrome have been proven to be valid. The most common theory is that chronic fatigue syndrome is caused by viral infection. After a viral infection, fatigue or tiredness can persist for some time. The flu virus can cause fatigue, which lasts for several weeks after the other symptoms have gone.

Most viral infections are gone within one week. Even though there is no evidence that a person has an enduring infection there are no explanations for why symptoms persist. Chronic fatigue can be caused by viruses, but researchers are still unsure if this is possible. The condition can also be made worse by recurring infections caused by bacterial germs or other viruses.

Inadequate immune system

It can affect almost all health conditions. Chronic fatigue syndrome is characterized by a weak immune system, according to studies. Stress, too much activity, and a sedentary lifestyle are all factors. Poor diet and pollution can be factors. Mixed results have been found regarding the immune system of individuals and their relationship to the syndrome.

Researchers have come up with the hypothesis that chronic fatigue syndrome could be caused by a viral infection that causes the production of cytokines.

CFS patients may have immune complexes, but related tissues have been damaged. This is a sign of an autoimmune disease. Although not all patients with CFS have allergies, secondary illnesses and allergic diseases may also play a role. Patients were more likely to be sensitive to certain foods, medications, and alcohol.

Hormonal imbalance

Some people with this syndrome have experienced blood levels abnormalities that their hypothalamus caused. This is not yet clear. Stress, age, and sex are all risk factors. It affects mostly people between the ages of 40 and 50. Statistics show that this syndrome is more common in women. The syndrome can also be caused by stress.

Tiredness and fatigue can indicate a psychological disorder or infection. If you have cognitive problems or chronic fatigue, seek medical attention.

Who is at risk?

According to statistics, America is home to more than 1 million people suffering from chronic fatigue syndrome. This condition has affected more people than lupus and sclerosis combined. Researchers continue to search for potential risk factors and causes of CFS. There are many unknowns about CFS. However, there are some common indicators that indicate risk.

Although the syndrome is more common in women, it can also be seen in men. While it is less common in children younger than adults, the disease is more common in adolescents and adults. It can also occur in people of different races and ethnicities, but it is less common among Hispanics or African Americans than it is among Caucasians. It can sometimes be seen in family members, but it is not contagious. Experts believe that there is a genetic connection. Further research is needed.

The Classification Controversy

CFS is a long-term and chronic neurological condition that the World Health Organization has identified. However, it is still not fully accepted by the medical community. The guidelines set forth by WHO are not supported by the National Institute of Health and Care Excellence (NICE) group of health professionals. In 2011, almost 85% of British Neurologists declared that chronic fatigue syndrome could not be classified as a neurological condition.

It is also difficult to diagnose chronic fatigue syndrome. After other conditions have been ruled out, a doctor should confirm the diagnosis. Different health organizations have basic guidelines for diagnosing the condition.

Chapter 5: How to Identify the Factors That Lead To Burnout

The human body and mind are capable of great things but they also have limitations. Each person has their own unique strengths and weaknesses, which essentially determine what they can achieve. These limits are usually ignored, but we learn ways to overcome them over time. Sometimes, some limitations can even be negligible. What happens if you break these limits?

You get burnt out. Exercising excessive amounts of stress can cause burnout. Burnout is when you are unable to cope with stressful situations and lose your motivation to do so. This is a serious condition which can affect your physical, mental and emotional well-being.

There are several factors that can cause burnout in the workplace. These are the most common:

Continuous pressure to achieve target goals. You are expected to perform at your best in every job. As with everything in high-pressure environments, you will burn out if your expectations are unrealistic or unreasonable.

Uncertainty regarding your job security. The global economy suffered a severe blow after the 2008 financial crisis and has yet to recover fully from it. Many companies resort to budget cuts and reorganizations that ultimately lead to layoffs. Fear of being next on the cutting block can cause anxiety and stress in your mind and heart. You can add on the additional responsibilities and duties left behind by those who were not able to keep their jobs and you have an extra workload.

Inability to handle increasing tasks. If your energy level isn't sufficient to cope with the workload, you become overwhelmed with stress and lose the ability to adapt. This can be worsened if you lack motivation, such as a sense of fulfillment, happiness, financial or tangible incentives, to keep you going.

It's easy to tell if you have burnout. These are the classic symptoms of burnout.

Extreme exhaustion. It is normal to feel exhausted on certain days. Chronic exhaustion is a different story. You may be exhausted if you feel constantly tired to the point where it is difficult to get out of bed each morning.

Resignation from social interactions with family and friends. You may withdraw from your friends and family, or find excuses to be alone. This happens especially to people who were once socially connected but now find themselves disinterested or quiet. You don't see the value of socializing and prefer to retreat to your own corner.

Inability to focus. It's possible to not get things done because you're either not interested or you don't have the ability to focus because you want to escape it all.

You lack the energy or enthusiasm to get things done. It's easy to drift aimlessly because you don't have the energy or enthusiasm to get out of this situation. This is when you stop caring about what the future holds or what others think.

Inability to fall asleep. It is becoming increasingly difficult to fall asleep at night due to the negative thoughts in you head.

Chronic body pains. You may feel persistent pain in your stomach, spine, and head along with exhaustion. Even after you take medication, the pain does not disappear.

As a way to deal with the situation, you may resort to drugs and alcohol. These things can provide you with an escape from your current situation and a temporary high that is completely opposite to the feeling of helplessness.

Increased sense of helplessness. You believe that no one, not even yourself, can solve your problem. You lose interest in everything and you believe that you can't make a difference by changing your mind.

As with any other problem, acknowledging your burnout is the first step to overcoming it. It is not worth denying that it exists. It is in your best interests to seek treatment if you have any of the above symptoms.

If left unchecked burnout can lead to a variety of serious and debilitating effects that don't just affect you. Personally, you're at greater risk for mental and emotional imbalances, as well potential health problems. If you have been a victim to drugs or alcohol, you are more likely to stall your career or mismanage your finances.

You are putting your relationships at risk with your friends, family and colleagues. You can cause them to worry about you, or drift away from your family and friends if you don't engage enough with them. You can reduce the amount of interaction you have with them, which can affect the quality of your relationship.

Burnout is rooted in your inability to deal with stress. It is important that you review your current habits and find better ways to manage stress. Your ability to deal with stress can often make the difference between success or failure in your workplace. This chapter will provide a detailed description of how to manage stress.

Chapter 6: Eat Well To Get Well

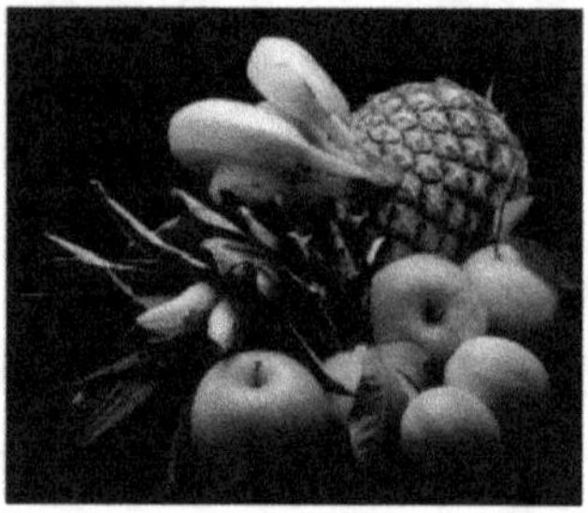

It's not just about sleeping in the bedroom, but also in your kitchen. Get a balanced breakfast and eat healthy meals throughout the day. Research shows that healthy whole foods, balanced meals and a healthy diet rich in carbs, protein and healthy fats can improve sleep quality. As we all know, the food you eat every day affects how your body functions. So it is natural that healthy wholefoods such as potatoes, rice and vegetables can provide your body with the vitamins and minerals it needs to enable the proper chemical processes to take place.

It's a good rule of thumb to remember that food should still look the same as its original form. Avoid processed foods, as they lack the vitamins and minerals that wholefoods provide. Multivitamins can be used to supplement vitamins you might have lost from your wholefood diet. Make sure you drink lots of water. Keep water bottles in your fridge, just like I do. It's practical and keeps you hydrated. You can also take it with you to work or carry it around.

There are many foods that naturally increase melatonin levels. GreenMedInfo reports that researchers from Thailand's Khon Kaen University discovered that certain tropical fruits can have significant effects on melatonin levels. Researchers gave the subjects a range of fruits, and measured the amount of melanin in the body using 6-sulfatoxymelatonins (aMT6s).

Researchers discovered that pineapples, oranges, and bananas could significantly increase melatonin levels. Pineapples significantly increased the amount of aMT6s by more than 266%, while bananas increased levels 180%. The ability to increase melatonin levels by around 47% was demonstrated by oranges. These can be eaten throughout the day to provide the body with the nutrients it needs to make melatonin at night.

Overview of Melatonin-Boosting Foods

* Pineapples.

* Bananas.

* Oranges

* Oats

* Sweet corn.

* Rice

* Tomatoes.

*Barley

Chapter 7: Love Myself

ELIXIRS OF LOYALITY

HARMONY IN A TINY BOOT

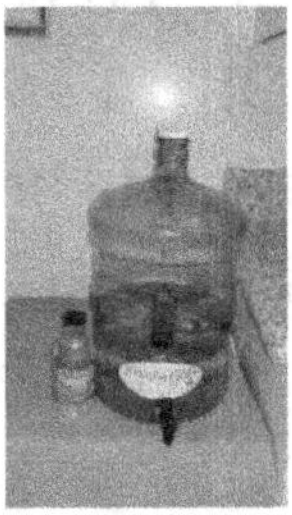

Our Ancient heritage includes Alchemy, Tinctures and Tinctures as well as Elixirs, Tinctures, Tinctures, Tinctures, and Elixirs. They were mentioned in Egypt's Bibles and in antiquity.

Stephen Salters, an incredible man who answered my questions and helped me create some ELIXIRS, was a wonderful person I met. Stephen displayed several hundred at The Conscious Life Expo Los Angeles, California.

These ELIXIRS are different in name and frequency, which allows us to address deeply rooted issues, problems, needs, and desires. Out of curiosity, I tried the sample. Stephen led me as I placed a few drops on my wrist. I felt a sense of calm and peace over my body within 3 to 5 minutes. For about 10 minutes, I didn't move. It was so peaceful and peaceful that I wanted to just sit there. I know that if I hadn't been in public places, even though he provided quiet areas for his customers to enjoy their company, I would have wept with joy. Although it's hard to describe the otherworldly feelings I experienced, I could not help but stay in this light for hours. It was amazing!

The ELIXIR was the right name for me because these were the areas where I experienced the most stress and difficulties in my life. Driving on L.A. freeways, going through airport security, and flying on planes. The law went into effect in two days, my friends. It was like a magic carpet opening on the freeway. I flew to work, and then I breezed through security at airport like magic. Because I spray it in the air prior to my flight, customers on board my plane felt instantly calmer and relaxed. Stephen was recommended by other flight attendants who noticed a significant difference in their moods after spraying some on their wrists. Happy passengers make for happy flight attendants who travel with ease and fun.

A friend of mine began using the mixture of bath salts and Elixirs Stephen made to help her lose weight. Within 4 to 5 days, she called me to inform me that she was getting up earlier and walking again. She was also losing weight slowly and easily. It was great. She thanked me repeatedly.

In the past two years, I have used different ELIXIRS as well as a few others during a detox that my adult son started. It was so much easier than using herbal formulas.

Visit Stephen's website and treat yourself. www.Elixirsoflove.com

Click on the following categories to choose your Elixirs. Ella the Author will greet you.

HYDRATE

You are what you eat.

Many of the poorest people in the world could be free from many diseases if they had access to clean water. This information is from my book:

According to the report, more than 350,000 people are affected by water-related diseases each year. Lack of safe water, sanitation, and hygiene remain one of the most pressing health problems in the world.

Although it may be hard to believe, not all bottled water is the same. Many bottled water sold in stores is "dead", as they lack minerals. Most of the water we consume doesn't reach our cells. This means that most of the water we drink is not reaching our cells. Additionally, the average American diet is so acidic we require alkaline water in order to balance our pH.

www.youtube.com/ELLACRONEY/FOREVERYOUNG and watch the interview I had the privilege to do with Glen, the founder of PristineHydro. You can also watch the YouTube interview with my dentist, who used Pristine water in her house after reading my book. Within a week, the whole family noticed a change. All of them had more energy, increased full bowel movements, clearer skin, and clearer thinking.

Because I was always dehydrated, I started drinking Pristine water when I was a flight attendant. I drank two liters each day of bottled water. Every morning, I now drink two 16-ounce glasses of Pristine water and notice a difference in my health. I have shared Pristine water over the years with pilots and flight attendants. They were amazed at its effectiveness and continue to use it. After using Pristine water for two weeks, one of my clients was able not to take blood pressure medication anymore and another client required less dialysis treatment.

Others have also used Pristine water after major surgery to support them.

Pristine uses a 10-stage Filtration process and is currently the leader in this field with its unique, patent-pending, environmentally friendly filtration system.

This new standard in acid-free, high-alkaline drinking water is set by the advanced re-mineralization and restructuring, recharging and reprogramming processes.

They can ship water bottles to your home.

Contact Ginger or Glen at 1-949-581-9191, or visit

www.http://livepristine.myshopify.com/#_1_38

Tell Ella the Author that you sent it, and let's get to living.

Leslie and Tom, my friends, asked me to try 9.5 Kangen water. I loved it. I felt like I had a lot of oxygen and was able to read again without glasses. We now have healthier water options.

Call 1 (949) 415-5017 for more information.

SQUATTING - FOR HEALTH

As children, we all did this: sat on our little legs and held our knees. This simple position actually has many benefits.

Squatting is a great way to support your bladder and prevent leakage from occurring when you sneeze. When it happens in public, leakage can be quite embarrassing. According to chiropractors, squatting seals the ileocecal vessel, which is located between the colon and small intestine. You can also use your thighs to avoid straining while you go to the toilet.

Squatting increases muscle strength, quadriceps, hamstrings, and calves. It naturally releases testosterone and growth hormones. When squats are performed correctly, they provide an environment that is highly anabolic for other areas of the body to grow. Squatting is a great way to build muscle mass and strength all over your body.

Squats helps maintain balance. Mobility goes hand in hand with this. More strength can be achieved by creating balance. This applies to all compound lifts such as deadlifts and bent-over barbell rows. Push presses for the upper body are also possible. This will provide balance and support for lower body lifts like leg presses, single-leg lunges, and single-leg squats. Squats are possible anywhere.

You can do squats at home or in the gym. They are the perfect exercise that you can do anywhere. You don't need to be a member or have expensive equipment like 20-30 reps of bodyweight squats or prisoner squats. These can be done at home, in the gym, at the beach, or in the park as part of cross-training.

Let's make it safe and minimize injuries. This will ensure that you have a more enjoyable experience. Here's a step-by-step guide to performing the basic squat exercise.

Keep your head straight. Your head should face forward. Your chest should be open.

Place your feet on a level surface. Place your feet shoulder-width apart.

Relax your arms and reach forward like a mummy. Relax.

Slowly lower your head into a sitting position. This is done by pressing your weight onto the heels. Your back is straight. Now, get back to your original standing position.

Your butt should be lowered so that your thighs are parallel to the ground. Your knees should reach directly above your ankles.

Tip: For beginners, it's a good idea for a chair to be placed directly behind you. When you lower into a squat position, your butt should touch the chair's outermost portion. This is your cue to get back up. Voila!

Chapter 8: Probable Causes

Although the cause of Fibromyalgia remains unknown, there are many factors that can trigger its onset. These include viral or bacterial infections, hyperthyroidism, lupus, rheumatoid, and hyperthyroidism. These triggering events may not be the primary cause of Fibromyalgia, but they can trigger the physiological abnormality. The related abnormalities include dysfunction in the immune system and sleep disturbances, hormone irregularities, mental fatigue, elevated substance and nerve growth, and hormonal irregularities.

Fibromyalgia can also manifest as muscle cramps and weakness. This disease can affect anyone, including children. Fibromyalgia is more common in women than it is in men. According to statistics, around 1/4 of those affected are unable work because of the fluctuating chronic symptoms.

Research has shown that stressors such as environmental, emotional, and physical can cause symptoms to worsen. Fibromyalgia can be triggered by undue stress.

Fibromyalgia can be referred to as a syndrome because of the numerous symptoms and related health conditions. Fibromyalgia is most commonly associated with pain in the muscles, ligaments, and tendons. This is why patients feel all over the body ache. It was described as feeling pulled or overworked. According to the prognosis, the symptoms can have a significant impact on daily life. Fibromyalgia can also be disabling and life-threatening.

What could trigger Fibromyalgia symptoms?

Although experts are still unsure of the cause, they do consider other factors such as genetics and infections. Experts are trying to find a genetic mutation that could make it more likely that a person will get the disease. This is how genetic predispositions can lead to Fibromyalgia.

Fibromyalgia can be triggered by certain health conditions. Fibromyalgia can also be linked to post-traumatic stress disorder.

Substance P

Recent studies have revealed new information about Fibromyalgia. One is that Fibromyalgia sufferers experience pain differently. Fibromyalgia sufferers have three times more CSF (cerebro-spinal fluid) than those without the condition. CSF is responsible to transmit pain impulses from our brain. Most likely, this will cause intense pain.

Insufficient deep sleep

Others believe that inadequate deep sleep could be the cause of the disease. The stage 4 phase of the sleep cycle is when our muscles are able to recover from the day's activities and then rejuvenate themselves. Fibromyalgia sufferers tend to experience a more light sleep once they reach stage 4. Even if they are sleeping for a long time, they suffer from poor quality sleep. Researchers invite normal volunteers to participate in an experiment. These volunteers were not allowed to enter stage 4 of sleeping. They also experienced similar symptoms to Fibromyalgia patients.

Functional Medicine:

Functional medicine addresses the root causes of chronic conditions such as Fibromyalgia. Conventional medicine treats only pain management. This type of medicine treatment believes that the disease is caused in part by the following:

Candida is a yeast or fungal infection that lives in the intestines. Candida overproduction can cause damage to the intestinal walls and perforate the bloodstream. It will release toxic byproducts into the body, which can lead to a variety of health problems, including fatigue, pain, and brain fog.

Gluten intolerance - This has been linked with chronic diseases. It is often called the "big maskader". Most symptoms of gluten intolerance do not involve digestive issues, but are neurological. This includes cognitive impairments, fatigue, pain and behavioral issues as well as depression.

Gluten can cause leaky gut and SIBO (small bacterial overgrowth) This can then lead to food intolerances, which is a vicious circle.

Thyroid disorders - These symptoms are also known as Fibromyalgia. To ensure that the thyroid glands function accurately, it is important to have your blood markers checked regularly.

Mycotoxins - toxic substances made from molds that functional medicine practitioners believe can trigger Fibromyalgia.

Vitamin deficiencies - vitamin deficiencies are the most common among people and can trigger the disease.

Chronic stress can cause adrenal fatigue. Our adrenal glands are stressed by intense pain. Food intolerances are often the first stressor. It can also be caused by mercury, toxicity and Candida overgrowth.

Other Factors

All of the causes mentioned above are interrelated. Fibromyalgia is not a common root cause. Although it isn't clear why Fibromyalgia develops more in women than men, there are many factors that you can take into consideration.

Atypical pain - One of the most popular theories is that Fibromyalgia sufferers develop changes in their central nervous system's ability to process pain messages. Chemical changes can cause this. The central nervous system, which includes the brain and nerves as well as the spinal cord, transmits all information to the body using specialized cells. Fibromyalgia is a condition that causes extreme pain sensitivity.

Fibromyalgia can be caused by disturbed sleep - As mentioned, insufficient sleep or disturbed sleeping patterns could trigger Fibromyalgia. This condition can also lead to fatigue. The disease can also be caused by sleep problems.

Chemical Imbalance – Some research has shown that Fibromyalgia sufferers have low levels in hormones like serotonin, noradrenaline, and dopamine. These hormones are thought to be a major factor in the onset of the disease. These hormones are essential in the regulation of one's appetite, mood, and sleep in response stressors. These hormones play an important role in the brain's ability to interpret pain signals from the nerves. A medication that increases hormone levels can disrupt pain signals.

There is no cure for this chronic condition, but there are many medications and treatments that can help the patient manage the symptoms.

Chapter 9: The Truth about Fats, Proteins and Carbs

Over the years, there have been many opinions about what is healthy food. The idea that people should eat low-fat and high-carbohydrate foods was popularized in the middle of the 20th century. When it came to weight loss, fat was considered to be the enemy. Carbohydrates were viewed as your source of endless energy. The American Heart Association as well as The American Dietetic Association were major supporters of the low-fat, high-carb diet. Modern scholars such as Dr. Michael and Mary Eades and Dr. Barry Sears rewrote the low-fat/lose-weight theory. Sears wrote the book entitled. It was initially intended for cardiologists but became more popular with mainstream readers. According to his book, the best way to eat healthy is to balance carbohydrates, fats, and proteins. This ratio should be 40% carbs to 30% protein and 30% fats in your daily diet. Low-carbohydrate diets are criticized by Sears and low-fat diets are praised as having too many carbohydrates. However, the ideal diet for healthy insulin and glucose levels is a low-carbohydrate diet.

Sears' diet may contain a lot of carbs. However, contrary to what many health experts believe, carbs are essential for the body to function properly. Low-fat diets are not ideal for weight loss and energy. Many studies, such one by The State University of New York Buffalo, show that a low-fat diet can lead to poor health. This includes a weak immune system and lower calcium intake.

It's difficult to understand that there is so much conflicting information. When I started to read the books about good nutrition, I was overwhelmed by all the differing opinions. One doctor says carbs are dangerous, and another one claims fat is the culprit. I was compelled by each one to think the way they did until the next theory came along. I have long since deciphered the truth from this mess of mixed beliefs. You may already know this, but each piece of advice on healthy food choices is true.

You are likely to be aiming for weight loss and energy boost if you're reading this book. The best way to eat all three components of your diet is to include them: fats, carbohydrates, and proteins. It is important to eat healthy fats and the right type of carbohydrates.

People who hate carbs might try to tell people that they are bad. It is impossible to be more truthful. Carbohydrates are basically sugar molecules in chains. Sugar molecules are made up of three components: carbon, hydrogen, and oxygen. We now have the scientific definition. Here is the popular belief that carbs are bad. Your digestive system attempts break down carbohydrates into single sugar molecules so they can be absorbed into your bloodstream. Fiber, which is not fully digestible, is one example of a carb that cannot be broken down. However, we will return to fiber later as it's a separate category. The cars that are easy to digest are converted into glucose, also called blood sugar. The glucose you consume is stored in your fat cells, while the rest is converted into energy. Your insulin can fluctuate quickly if you have carbs stored as glucose. This is true for fast-burning carbs. These are the carbs to avoid. These carbs are easy to digest by your metabolism. This can cause your insulin and glucose levels to crash, which will not be in your best interest when it comes time for weight loss or energy boosting. These carbs can increase your energy within minutes. However, this burst of energy can be short-lived and almost always follows by an energy crash. These fast-burning carbs make up your breakfast pastries (yes even blueberry muffins), baked potatoes, and candy bars. These carbs can be hard to live without, especially if you're trying to lose weight or boost your energy.

Slow-burning carbs should be avoided. Your body requires them for proper functioning. Because they contain longer and more complex chains of sugar molecules, these carbs are harder to digest. Slow-burning carbs are found in most vegetables, fruits, and whole grains. These carbs move through your bloodstream slower, which allows glucose to peak slowly and more evenly. This allows your insulin to perform its task properly. Your insulin is responsible for distributing glucose to your cells, either to store it in fat cells or burn it as fuel. Slow-burning carbs slow down the rate at which your glucose rises, instead of rapidly peaking. Although this gradual increase will not give you an instant energy boost, it is more noticeable than the one after eating a cookie (fast burning carb), it will allow you to maintain the energy and distribute it evenly. You'll feel more energetic throughout the day after eating a piece fruit than after munching on two donuts. You're probably thinking, "Two doughnuts!" I've never had two doughnuts! You might want to do this, even though you may not choose the second doughnut. I can guarantee you will opt for a similar "satisfying" food such as pizza slices, iced tea, and so on. Because you can never have enough of a quick-burning carb. It's necessary to have another one within a short time. It will feel like you are running on empty.

When they said that fat is what makes you "fat", the well-meaning health professionals of yesteryear thought very rationally. They were wrong, however. The Harvard School of Public Health reports that only 13% of Americans were considered obese in 1960, when Americans ate approximately 45% of their calories from fats and oil. Today, 34% of Americans are obese. However, our caloric intake from fats and oils has fallen to 33%.

What went wrong? What went wrong? The food was still delicious even though fat was removed from the equation. To make the low-fat food more appealing, you can add sugar, salt, and processed grains. It turned out to be less nutritious than it was. Artificial sugar, salt, and other chemicals only promote obesity and chronic diseases. As if that weren't enough, your body does need some types of fat. By sticking to a diet that doesn't include fat, you can effectively eliminate both the good and bad fats. It's easy. Saturated fats can be bad for your health. They contribute to diabetes, heart disease, and other related diseases. Monounsaturated and polyunsaturated oils are the exact opposite. They help your heart function, as well as other parts of your body.

Fat is your best source of energy, and it's true. It acts as a firewall between your cells, determining what enters and leaves them. Many vital vitamins and minerals that your body produces are based on cholesterol. Fats are not soluble but can be mixed with water or blood. Fat particles can travel through bloodstreams in either small, dense, or thick forms. HDL (High Density Lipoproteins), a form of cholesterol that your body can benefit, is a good choice. Your doctor will tell you to avoid the bad cholesterol.

Good cholesterol is not the only important type of fat you can consume daily, especially if your goal is to increase your energy and reduce inflammation. I will talk more about those fats, particularly Omega 3 fatty acid, later. But for now let's look at protein and the reasons you need it to boost your energy and lose weight. Protein is closely related to fat in that almost all foods containing protein also contain fatty acids. A protein is a long chain of amino acids. An amino acid is a chemical composition made up of hydrogen, oxygen and nitrogen. Although your body can produce proteins by itself, it only has 14 of the 22 types of amino acid to use. The 8 remaining essential amino acids can be obtained from protein-rich food. Each of these 22 amino acids has a unique function that works in your favor. All of these amino acids promote energy and weight loss. Even though proteins do not directly boost energy, the fact that they maintain different parts of the body is an important factor that can affect your energy levels.

There has never been a convincing argument against protein; in fact, they are good for you. That's it. There has been much written about foods that are high in protein. People who live a low-fat lifestyle discourage eating protein at every meal. Protein is usually found in foods that are high in fat. It is well-known that protein should be consumed with every meal. This holds true when it comes to gaining energy.

"Okay, all this information is great. But what should I eat?"

You were sure to ask.

You could simply avoid all processed foods, I could say. This was all I had to do at first. This is great advice and something that every health professional would endorse. If you are looking to lose weight while simultaneously increasing your energy, then read on.

Chapter 10: Exercise

Exercise is a great way to boost your mood and energy. You'll see a rise in your energy levels and be able to maintain them if you do regular exercise. Exercise not only gives you more energy but also releases stress and makes you feel happier. Additionally, you'll have more energy to get through the day.

To get a great workout, you don't need to spend a lot or do fancy exercises. It doesn't take a lot of work to get a good workout. You can do a simple walk around the neighborhood or to a park for 10-20 minutes per day. You can also exercise during work if you don’t have the time. You can take the stairs, instead of the elevator, park further away from your office or grocery store and walk more. If you are able, walk to work instead. There are many creative ways to get your exercise in throughout the day. These are some of the ideas I have created to get your creative juices flowing, and to motivate you to exercise.

* Spend 10 minutes each morning dancing to your favorite tunes

* Take advantage of the weekend to try different classes at your gym.

* You can jump on a trampoline every day for between 10-20 minutes. This is similar to jumping rope, and you can burn lots of calories. It's also super fun.

* Go roller skating or ice skating;

* Invite your family members to join you in your exercise program, or your friends.

You can enjoy the great outdoors by riding your bike around the neighbourhood or along a trail.

* Do small exercises while watching T.V. or work out at home while watching a movie.

* Reintroduce a childhood favourite and hula hoove your way to greater energy and better health.

* Reward yourself for reaching a milestone.

You don't need to find exercise difficult, exhausting, or overwhelming. It's up to you to choose the right exercise for you. You can also personalize your workout to suit your needs. You will need to be motivated to move your body, especially if it has been sitting there for a while. These are some motivational tips to help you get moving again.

* Track your progress with computer or phone apps

* Purchase good-looking, functional workout clothes that will motivate you to wear and use them.

* Keep a fitness log and track your exercise routines regularly.

Find inspiration online to help you stay motivated. For example, find an image of your ideal body.

To motivate yourself to exercise every day, join an online community.

* Check out these fitness success stories.

* Make a list of the reasons you exercise. Include energy and fatigue! •

* Read books on health and fitness.

Inspiration is everywhere. You can find it all around you to inspire you to stay fit and prevent fatigue, improve your health and look better.

Chapter 11: Liver Support

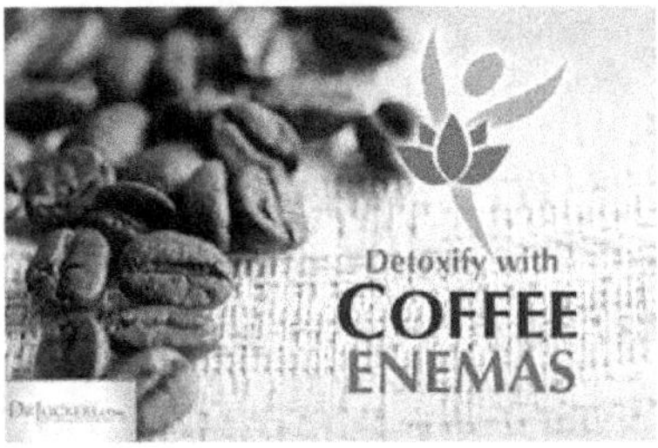

You may do coffee enemas if you are

CBS Upregulator

Crohn's Disease can make it difficult to drink coffee enemas. Coffee enemas are my first choice for liver support. Since the moment I found out I had MCS I purchased "Wellness Against All Odds" by Sherry Rodgers, M.D. I used to do a coffee enema every day.

Many people find it hard to imagine any kind of enema. Coffee enemas are known to have been around for many years. They were actually included in the Merck Manual until 1977.

Detoxifying can cause you to feel ill, nauseous and achy. You can eliminate toxic waste quicker with coffee enemas. You are no longer a back-up, in my opinion.

What does a coffee enema do?

The caffeine in coffee circulates through hemorhoidal veins in its rectum to the enterohepatic and portal systems, where it reaches the liver via the portal vein.

The portal vein forces toxic bile out of the body and into the gut. The caffeine stimulates the production of glutathione-S-transferase, which is important in making glutathione. I will now discuss in detail how Glutathione is used as a major conjugator for Phase II detoxification.

There are two phases to detoxification.

Phase I and Phase 2. People who are chemically sensitive usually have Phase I that is fast and Phase II that is normal or slow. If Phase I is rapid, it can produce a chemical such as formaldehyde that is many times more toxic than its original compound. Glutathione supports Phase II. It adds another molecule to make the toxin less toxic. It would be wonderful to bind toxic bile that is being released from the liver into your intestines. Use your BIND. You can substitute activated charcoal, clay or zeolite if you have an allergy to BIND

Did you know that coffee enemas can be used even if you have an allergy to it? Dr. Sherry Rogers sure did! I've heard from some people that they don't like the smell. You can use an electric burner to brew your coffee outside.

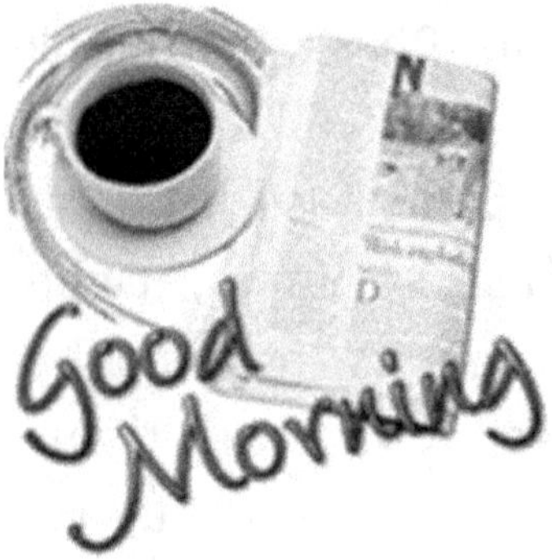

My modified coffee enema method will remove the caffeine-induced high if you've tried a coffee enema before and got sick or buzzed from it.

My modified instructions for coffee enemas have proven to be very effective.

I do mine every morning!

Modified coffee enema available for patients with CHRONIC Illness

What you will need: A checklist

* BIND

* Magnesium Chloride Solutions

* Organic Coffee (except Cafe Altura).

* Kit for glass or stainless steel enema buckets

* A ceramic or glass pot is used to make coffee (not stainless steel).

* Small mesh strainer made of stainless steel.

* Bodyceuticals Calendula Salve and Unpetroleum Jelly

* Disposable Nitrile – Latex-free gloves available at any Walgreens.

* A step stool for the bathroom. Amazon.com:

How to prepare your body

* Take B.I.N.D. 30 minutes prior to enema

Take 1 teaspoon Magnesium Chloride Solution in 6-8oz. water.

* This will allow for relaxation of muscle tissue, allowing for easy release.

* Eat slowly so you don't become weak. Some prefer to have a bowel movement

prior to doing the coffee enema. For me, this was impossible. It was possible when I wanted.

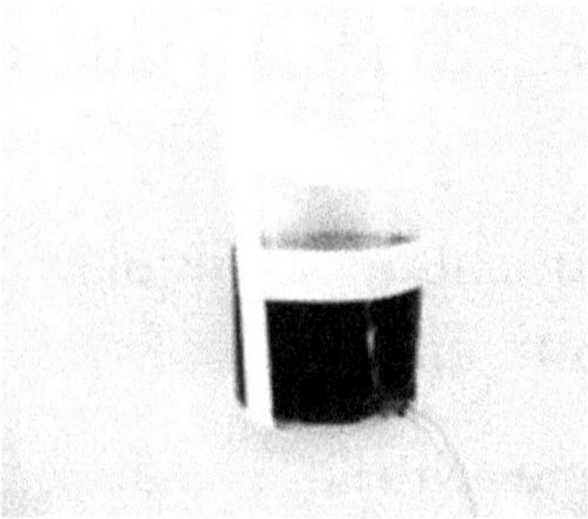

Making coffee

The coffee solution will be made into 4 cups. Each cup will be broken down into 2 cups. Two cups of coffee solution must be used to make a complete enema. Then, two cups should be removed and then another 2 cups must be added and released.

Bring 2 cups of water to a boil

Mix 3 tablespoons organic coffee in a bowl and stir it into the mixture.

* Reduce the temperature to a low simmer and let it simmer for 20 minutes.

* Take the pot off the stove.

2. Add 2 cups of hot water to your coffee

Now you will have four cups of coffee at a roughly lukewarm temperature, ready to use immediately. You can add some ice cubes to cool it down if it's still too hot.

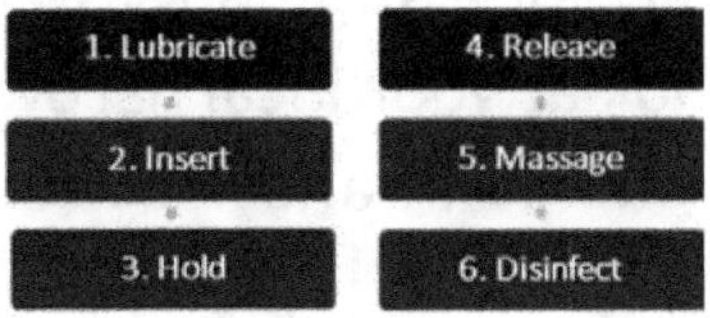

* Strain the coffee into a strainer and pour it into two cups

* Fill the Pyrex with 2 cups of coffee and take it to the bathroom.

* Assemble the bucket, tubing, and rectal tip.

You should close the clamp first to prevent coffee stains from getting on your bathroom floors. It has happened to me many times!

* Add two cups of coffee from the Pyrex glass measuring cup to the bucket.

* Use the hook included with your enema set to hang it from a towel rail in your bathroom.

*If the size of the hook included in the kit is too small, you can improvise and buy a larger S hook at your local hardware store. Hang the enema in a low place. It should not be hung from a showerhead or a shower rod.

* Hang the enema bucket from the towel rack.

* Lay a towel on the ground. I use a brown towel. LOL!

* Keep the Calendula Salve and Unpetroleum jelly close by.

Now you are ready to go!

The 6 Step Modification

coffee enema technique

The First Half (500ml or 2 cups).

Allow enough coffee solution to flow from the enema bucket, allowing for a free flow of liquid without any air bubbles entering the rectum. To dump it, you can use the toilet bowl. To account for the coffee solution, add water to the bucket.

Step 1. Step 1.

* Take the rectal end of the enema tube and apply the Calendula Salve or Unpetroleum jelly to it. [Use "Preparation H" because it contains Mercury, "Vaseline", or "KYJlly" instead. Both contain petroleum.

Step 2. Step 2.

* Place the rectal enema tip on your left side.

* Unclamp tubing, allowing a small amount of coffee solution to get in. Each

time you feel the urge to go, take the enema tip from your rectum and wait several seconds.

Continue to insert until the coffee solution is nearly gone. Due to the bucket's design, some coffee may remain in it.

Step 3. Step 3.

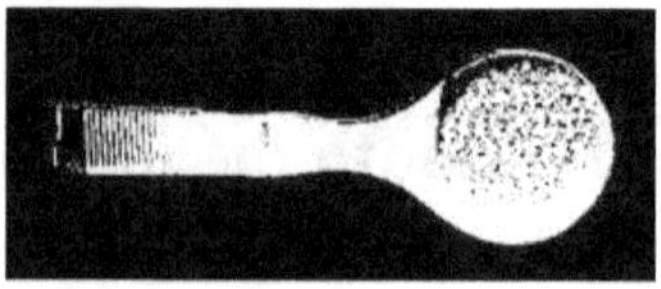

* It may be necessary to hold the tip or tube in your hand so it doesn't fall from your anus.

* Your body will soon learn to retain the coffee solution for long enough to make it effective.

For 10-15 minutes, you should hold 2 cups of coffee.

Fifteen minutes is preferred. It's the time you keep it there that is important, not the amount of coffee you add. It feels daunting at first.

Be patient! Practice makes perfect.

Step 4. Step 4.

Place your stepstool in the toilet. After 15 minutes, flush the coffee in the toilet. Although I am unable to send photos, I do take the seat off the toilet and place my feet on the rim. The enema solution is then released. Don't forget, I was not very overweight when I started coffee enemas. It was simple.

When I was in Paris, France with my boyfriend, I was looking for a place to go to the bathroom. I found a lavatory. Surprised, I discovered a hole in the ground. I was shocked and ran for my life. "The toilet bowl is gone!" I shouted. People told us that there are bathrooms outside so that you can squat down and go!

Buy a footstool. They can be purchased online at Amazon.com. It is vital for proper evacuation.

Step 5. Rectal Massage

This is an important step that should not be overlooked. It is essential that you do this! You are more likely to become sick if you don't do it. You should not skip this step. This is the rectal massage. This step is often misunderstood. Your rectum is located inside your body. Your anus is where the entrance is.

• Release as much of the coffee solution as possible until it is no longer available.

* Get your disposable Nitrile gloves

* With your index finger, insert the catheter into your rectum (where the tip was).

* Start to rub the mucous membrane walls of the rectum for a long enough time to induce peristalsis.

You will be exposed to more toxic crap. I apologize for the language but very few people can do this right. This technique is essential. I've never met anyone who didn’t use it. If you're wired, you can skip this step. It is messy. Yes. It's worth it. It's so hard to believe!

People have said to me that they didn't believe it was possible for them to have any left. I remind them, "Just when you think your job is done, go back and do another massage."

Step 6. Step 6.

* Always wash your hands well. To scrub your cuticles and fingernails with a nailbrush,

* Try to make it a habit not to place your fingers in your mouth.

Use an 8-ounce squirt container filled with liquid soap to clean the silicone tubing.

Rinse with water.

* Dry thoroughly. Now you are ready to move on.

The Second Half (500ml or 2 cups)

You are now ready to perform the second half of the coffee enema. You should check the temperature of the remaining 2 cups of coffee in your pot. If it is too cold, heat it up to the desired temperature.

Continue Step 1,2,3,4, 5,6

* Clean the silicone tubing again using an 8-ounce squirt container filled with liquid soap. The soap should be sprayed into the tubing at both ends. Fill the tubing with water.

Let the tubing with soapy water rest for a while before you rinse it. To dry the tubing, hang it. Use a toothbrush and any disinfectant to clean your toilet bowl.

You will soon get the hang of it after a few days. The chemicals will start to appear and smell. It's true.

Congratulations! Congratulations! You are a Brave Soul.

You'll be among the lucky ones who get well quickly and experience minimal discomfort. This is an important tool for healing and detoxification.

Castor oil packs

Castor oil packs can be used to treat many conditions, including liver problems. Castor oil can be heated on cotton flannel or wool to act as a counterirritant. It can irritate the skin's surface and cause dilation of blood vessels.

A castor oil kit is available for your convenience. You can choose to have the kit come with either wool or cotton flannels. Castor oil may be included in the kit. If not, you can purchase it separately. The flannel cloth should not be reused. It was recommended that you refrigerate the flannel cloth and then use it again and again. The chemicals in the used flannel will reenter your system.

How to use a Castor Oil Package

The flannel cloth should be placed over the liver. Cut a piece or wrap of plastic one to two inches bigger than the flannel fabric. Put the flannel cloth into a warm, oily solution. Take some liquid out.

Prepare the area where you will lie. To prevent staining, place a large sheet of plastic and an old towel on the surface. Place the oil-soaked flannel on top of your liver. Placing a piece of plastic over the flannel cloth. Place a hot water bottle on the area. Cover the area with a second towel.

You can rest for up to two hours. To remove the oil from your skin, use a mixture of three tablespoons baking soda and one quart water.

Liver flush

A liver flush is not recommended at this time. It's too much for your adrenals. They are very effective, although I am sure that some people swear by them. However, many energy practitioners, including me, do not believe in them.

Dry skin brushing

It aids in detoxification. The exfoliation part is simple to understand. Dry skin brushing can be used to detox. It is similar in function to massage. This helps to move the lymph fluid into the lymph nodes by using light pressure and brushing in a direction that is gentle on the skin.

Dry skin brushing increases circulation and delivers oxygenated blood to the skin. This helps them do their jobs more effectively.

What's the best way to dry your skin?

You will first need a brush. These can be purchased at most health food stores. Vegetable-derived bristles are best. For those difficult to reach places like your back, a long handle is necessary.

Dry brushing stimulates the body and energizes it. Most practitioners recommend it to be done in the morning before your shower. However, you can do it at any time you like. Start by brushing your skin from your feet, working your way up to your legs. Next, move your midsection (front and rear) up and then across your chest. End your arms towards your armpits. People believe that the detox and circulatory booster helps with skin conditions such as acne and digestive problems.

Chapter 12: How long do you need to sleep? What are the sleeping problems and solutions for more energy daily?

It is crucial to ensure that you are able to relax comfortably and for a sufficient amount of time. The eight-hour sleep recommendation is a guideline, but the ideal amount of sleep or rest for each person will vary. Too much or too little sleep can cause exhaustion, and other health problems. As you age, your ideal amount of sleep or rest may change.

You can find out how much sleep or rest you need by doing a research. This involves tracing your sleeping hours until you wake up normally at the time of your morning alarm. An app called Sleepytime can help you determine how much sleep you have, based on the length of your rest periods. You'll feel more awake and alert if you wake up in the middle of strong rest periods than in the middle of one.

Get the best sleep possible by determining your ideal sleeping hours.

For greater health and well-being, it is important to get enough sleep. However, the eight hour rule can be different for each person. To find your optimal time to go to bed, you can do a study to determine when you wake up. Here's how.

What amount of rest/hours do you really require?

Eight hours is the common rule for what constitutes a full night of sleep. This is assuming that everyone can recall it. However, this principle is not unusual. Two studies, one at Wally Reed Research Institution and one at School of California, looked at a variety of sleepers. They found that even seven hours of relaxation per night can quickly add up to a large amount of sleep debt.

Although the research was published in 2003 after four years of hard work, most people still believe that five to six hours of sleep per night is sufficient to function without any problems. Although it is true that some people can manage it, most of us need eight hours of sleep every night. Anything less than this and we experience serious failures in attention, response time, and attention.

For two weeks, the members of the research team were examined in a controlled lab. The eight- or nine-hour rest period did not show any signs of reducing down. However, the four- and six-hour categories were found to have been affected to the point that they could be compared to being legally drunk at the end the two week interval. It is not superior to overusing Saturdays or Sundays. You don't need to sleep more.

Research shows that adults who sleep between 6-7 hours a night have lower rates of death. Here are some ways to relax if you have trouble negotiating your eight-time allowance.

A third of the day should be spent sleeping, relaxing and charging for the next day. Research from the Nationwide Sleep Base shows that nearly a third of Americans wake up feeling tired, with almost the same number awakening in the morning. 21% of Americans wake up too early, and then have difficulty getting to sleep or having trouble sleeping.

What are the alternatives to getting frequent energy?

It's important to recognize that lack of sleep can be a serious problem.

Insomnia

According to NSF, insomnia is Latin for "no sleep", and it is the most common problem with rest in America. People come to the hospital regularly for help with sleeping.

Solutions

* Give your mind the necessary alerts to wake up when it's shining and wind down when it gets darker

* Dimm the lights at least 3 hours before bedtime

Limit caffeinated beverages to mornings

* If possible, shift the most traumatizing projects from the previous work day

Monkey Brain

It is one sign of sleeplessness that it takes you a long time to fall asleep. However, this is a unique problem that can make sleeping difficult, if not impossible.

Resting is an inactive act, so it can often backfire.

Solutions

* Do something that will allow you to rest before bed or after waking up

* Quiet the mind

* Try sound recordings or strong rest mobile applications

* Remember that it is better to be tired than to relax.

Snoring

Although snoring can be frustrating for those who are paying attention, it can also indicate sleep apnea which is a serious medical condition.

Solutions

* see a physician

* Inhale right strips

* Treat your principal enhancement procedure as a therapy

* If you are a person, go to bed before your partner.

It's difficult to get and it feels refreshing

Evening owls can make it difficult to sleep at night. Late sleep-phase disorder (DSPS), is a healthcare term that refers to a serious problem in the moment of sleep. DSPS can cause difficulty relaxing after a long night, and then you may have trouble getting up in the morning.

Solutions

* Do the distressing factor and wake up by opening the curtains

* Brighten the lighting and blare alarms

* Low satisfaction in bed is a similar crack that can help you wake up more easily

After several weeks of this painful exercise, you will be able to modify your behavior and become more aware of the time.

It's not only how much sleep you get, but also how good you sleep. Your sleep quality will be compromised if you wake up every hour or turn your head to the night. Many people with apnea have no idea they are suffering from it. These are some things you can do to improve your sleep quality:

* Rest monitoring technology can be used to help you determine how relaxed you really are.

* It is also possible to practice essential sleep hygiene (eliminate electronic devices after dark, avoid alcohol, and stop drinking caffeinated beverages, etc.). To ensure a better night's sleep.

* Keep your routine intact every day, even on weekends.

Chapter 13: How much sleep is enough?

To be fully rested, many people need to sleep between 7 and 9 hours each night. Some people can manage with seven to nine hours a night, while others need more.

As we age, the amount of sleep that an individual requires each night changes. While everyone has different sleep needs, the chart below shows the general recommendations for all age groups.

Age	The amount of sleep
Infants from 4-12 Months	Daily, 12-16 hours (including naps).
Children aged 1-2 years	11-14 hours daily (not including naps).
Children aged 3-5 years	10- 13 hours per day (including naps).
Children 6-12 Years	9-12 hours daily

Teenagers aged 13-18	8-10 hours daily
Adults aged 18 and over	7-8 hours daily

The loss of sleep can increase if you are losing sleep frequently or sleep less than the recommended amount. The sleep debt is the amount of sleep you lose. If you lose two hours each day, your total sleep debt will be approximately 14 hours over the course of a week.

Napping is a common way to deal with sleepiness. Napping does not give you the ability to sleep well at night. You may experience a temporary boost in alertness or performance. You cannot use napping as a way to replace lost sleep hours.

Many people spend more time sleeping on their days off than they do on their workdays. It could be an indicator that you aren't getting enough sleep. Even if you feel more rested on the days that aren't paid, it can impact your body's sleep-wake cycle.

Your health can be affected by long-term sleep loss and bad sleeping habits. Use a sleep diary to track your sleep habits and ensure you get enough. You can record how much sleep you get, how alert you feel, and how tired you feel when you wake up. Also, note how tired you feel at night.

Chapter 14: Extreme self care: Nourishing your Soul To Reduce Stress & Burn Out & Fatigue

Outrageous Self-Care means settling for decisions that honor your spirit in every day of your life.

Wendy, a customer of mine (her name has been changed), is an extremely productive originator. She felt overwhelmed, under-subscribed, unhappy, and constantly being beaten by her wealthy customers. I asked her to focus on extraordinary self-care and she replied, "Iris that is too essential." It's like telling a planner that she needs texture.

Wendy refocused her life on Extreme Self Care. She set higher standards, focused on the important things in her life, and made a list of everything she needed to do. Her life became a lot more pleasant. Wendy is a busy woman with a lot to do. She has lots of customers, money and work. She encouraged her customers to approach Wendy with respect and let them know that her flawless manifestations would be completed in no time. She began her adoration life all over again, and also made sure to take the time to walk, think and have fun.

Sometimes the rudiments can be exactly what we need to balance. It's difficult to see the difference between knowing what supports us and doing those brain, body, and soul things that bring you over into balance.

Being Your Best Self

Self care is the love you give yourself to be your best selves.

It is worth looking at all the options for self-care:

* Stress Elimination

* Environment

* Family

* Love Relationships

* Health

* Emotional Balance

* Ingestion: Water, food, drinks, vitamins, and so on.

* Appearance

* Daily Rituals

* Spiritual Practices

* Work Life Self Kindness: Bringing your best self to life

Extraordinary Self-Care in real life

Now it is your turn. Have a look at the thoughts that were recorded before. Choose 2-3 thoughts that you feel most strongly this week. Let's say you choose: Stress Elimination, Emotional Balance, and Appearance.

Now, for each classification, list 10 things you would find great comfort in the event you did those things.

Here's an example:

Passionate Balance:

1) Take a look at what I am currently focusing on. 2) If my thoughts are angry, pitiful or stress-inducing, choose the most inspiring musings to replace those feelings. ; 3) Talk to a friend and ask them for support, guidance and genuine help. 4) Go for a walk in the woods at least three times a week; 5) Take some time to write down my feelings; 6) Get me moving; 7) Allow my emotions to guide you. Respect and recognize what I feel. Simply be. ; 8) Set more solid limits to ensure that others don't "sludge me." ; 9) Have fun with my children. ; 10) I am open to love, joy, trust, and fun

Your Turn

Make Extreme Self Care a priority.

Do the following and enjoy the sensations of possibility, unwinding and joy. You can also use your adoring generosity as a way to bring out the best within yourself.

It is important to understand your blood type in order to improve your health and reduce your chances of developing immune system infections. Let's look at this concept in greater detail.

Many people take care to consider the type of blood they have. It is important when you are planning for an operation, or any other procedure that may require blood products.

Science has shown that blood classification is essential to reducing ailment or ailment, and for living a vibrant, solid life. A life that allows you to focus on your dreams, desires, and family, rather than visiting a specialist or healing center.

I was awarded accreditation in blood classification science (BT) by the Institute for Human Individuality. As of today, I am a member of a similar group. Following this preparation, I discovered the direct benefits of writing blood to create dietary suggestions.

Many people are familiar with ABO blood writing. There are four blood types: O, which accounts for 45% of the universe's population; A, which represents 40% of the total populace; B, which accounts for 11% of the global populace; and finally, AB, which only makes up 4%.

Your BT is determined by your family's genetic control. Your blood classification is only a small amount of sugar stuck to the outside of your red plateslet. Each cell in your body contains many different sugars, including blood classification sugars. Your DNA controls the sugars in your cells. Your blood classification, which is similar to eye or hair color, is a unique part of your identity. Your BT is the same regardless of whether you are AB or AB.

Fucose is the sugar for type O. Fucose will be mixed with N-Acetyl gallactosamine (or GalNac) for type A. Fucose and D-

Galactose make up the sort B sugar. Sort AB is a mixture of An and B with each of three blood classification sugars. This is why AB is the most common beneficiary of blood. Insusceptible framework distinguishes between what is "you", and what is not you. AB is able to perceive all three sugars and will not dismiss them. Sort O, also known as the all-inclusive benefactor, is the inverted. O blood does not have GalNac and D-Galactose. It sees all other blood types as "not me", and will try to pulverize them. Similar applies to B and A. They can both get blood from O but not each other.

Blood classifications do not only apply to individuals. Nature is full of sugars (antigens), which make up our blood classification. They are found in a variety of organisms and creatures. The infection is one example. D-galactose is used in many infections. D-galactose makes blood type B. This means that if someone is of sort B, the chance of them getting infected is greater. Similar to how a transfusion deals about "self" and "nonself", if you see an infection as if it were you (write B), then your body will be less likely to destroy it than if it was sort A. It is important to note that some nourishments also have blood classification antigens. Drain, which is rich in D-galactose (the type B sugar), is the best example of this. Another case is pork, which is a source of GalNac (the Type A sugar). Kelp is an important source of fucose which is the sugar for all blood types.

Additionally, sustenances contain substances called lectins that follow up on blood types to cause different changes in our bodies, such as, for instance, a change in our ability to absorb certain nutrients.

Make our plates stick together

Trigger vast aggravation

You can become insulin by connecting to insulin receptors in cells that prompt weight gain

Attack on the immune system

Pain and a trigger stomach-related framework glitch

Leaky Gut Syndrome is a condition that causes imagination to cause intestinal damage and mind irritation.

Interfere with nerve movements in the body and alter levels of neurotransmitters. This can lead to nerve and cerebrum destruction, and eventually Alzheimer's disease.

Joint aggravation can cause different types of joint pain.

Modify hormone levels and cause thyroid dysfunction

Chapter 15: Hypothyroidism Treatments

There are many treatments for hypothyroidism. One common treatment is to take daily hormone replacement tablets called levothyroxine. Your doctor will perform numerous blood tests to determine the right dosage for you.

The required amount of levothyroxine depends on the severity of the condition. It may take some time before you get the correct dose. Sometimes, it can take days to determine exactly how much. Patients are usually given lower doses initially and doctors then monitor how the body reacts to the hormone replacement tablets over time.

The dosage can be adjusted or decreased depending on how the body responds to it. Some patients may see miracles while others might not be able to get the desired results. You may see positive results immediately if you're lucky. Otherwise, it could take several months before you see any improvement.

Once you have determined the right dosage, your doctor will still require you to test your hormone levels once a year. Hypothyroidism can be a lifelong condition. You will need to depend on levothyroxine throughout your life. Patients are usually prescribed one tablet per day. To get the best results, it is recommended that patients take it with water and on an empty stomach. Do not take two pills later if you happen to miss a dose. We often believe we can simply take another pill to make up the missing dosage, but in reality medicines don't work that way.

Although levothyroxine can be a great solution for hypothyroidism it has its downsides. Side effects can occur when patients have hypothyroidism in its most severe stages and require a higher dose of levothyroxine. Side effects include chest pain, excess sweating, headaches and diarrhea. If you experience similar side effects to this treatment, talk with your doctor immediately.

You may also receive levothyroxine in combination with T3 (Triiodothyronine). This treatment can lead to serious conditions such as angina (excessive pain in your chest), arrhythmia (an irregular heartbeat), and osteoporosis (where bones weaken and degrade over time).

Patients who are pregnant should seek specialist care because there is a possibility that the baby could develop abnormally or have birth defects. Doctors will usually increase the dosage during this period to ensure that the baby is healthy.

Many factors play a major role in the success of these treatments. Your body's response to these treatments will depend on your age, diet, and any other medications. The effectiveness of treatments is usually determined by the patient's soy intake, body weight, gender, and iron supplement intake.

You now know the potential solutions to hypothyroidism. However, you also need to be aware of the side effects. Many patients prefer to heal naturally and avoid dependence on medication that could cause more severe illness. You can also live well with hypothyroidism naturally by reading the next page.

Chapter 16: Natural Pain Relief

Prescription medications may not work in certain circumstances. Sometimes, your body may not respond to certain treatments. It is important to avoid any allergic reactions, particularly pain relievers or anesthetics. Instead, you should consider natural pain relief options. The best healer is still nature. There are many herbs that have amazing healing properties. Here are some examples:

It is an active ingredient found in chili pepper. It temporarily reduces pain-prone nerve receptors by blocking C fibers. Capsaicin can be applied to the area injured and reduces the soreness for up to three to five weeks before the nerves feel normal again. Capsaicin has been shown to be effective and is available for sale in the United States. Capsaicin cream was reported to reduce arthritis pain by up to 50% in patients with arthritis after a month.

Both of these components can be found in holy basil, holy turmeric, and ginger. They are all anti-inflammatory agents. Turmeric is a natural pain reliever and is used in many delicious curries. Research has shown that turmeric may contain curcumin, which is known to ease inflammatory conditions such as rheumatoid and psoriasis. It has anti-cancer effects. Turmeric also aids in blood circulation and prevents the formation of blood clots. Curcumin reduces inflammation and pain by lowering the release of enzymes from damaged cells. It can be used to treat bruises, joint inflammation, skin, and digestive problems. The Chinese have used ginger to ease pain for thousands of years. It is used to relieve pain, such as nausea, headaches and menstrual cramps.

Valerian root is known as nature's tranquilizers. It helps to regulate the central nervous system, which can relieve anxiety, stress, insomnia, tension, irritability, mood swings, mood swings, and irritability. Valerian can be used to relieve pain by decreasing nerve sensitivity.

This component is commonly found in aspirins. It can also be found naturally in white willow barks. This pain relief is traditionally used to treat joint inflammation. Although white willow bark has a slower effect than commercial aspirin, it lasts much longer. White willow bark is not as irritating to the stomach as aspirin and doesn't cause any damage to the gastro-intestinal lining. White willow bark can also reduce the severity of migraine attacks, according to research.

Arnica, a component found in European flowers, is active. Although its healing mechanism is not known, it does have anti-inflammatory properties. This can be used to treat acute injuries or swelling following surgery. Painful swelling can be reduced by taking oral homeopathic arnica following surgery.

Tonic or herbal oils such as peppermint oil, camphor, eucalyptus and fennel can be used to treat normal headaches or migraines. You can apply them topically to the affected area. Their cooling and menthol properties help reduce inflammation and pain. Prostaglandin, a powerful agent that reduces inflammation, is made from digested fish oils. A study found that cod-liver oil was able to reduce NSAIDS use by up to 40% in patients with rheumatic arthritis. After 10 weeks of cod-liver fish oils, two-thirds of patients who suffer from neck and back pains were able stop taking NSAIDS.

MSM is an active ingredient of sulfur that prevents cartilage and joint degeneration. Scientists at the University of California, San Diego reported that osteoarthritis patients who were treated with MSM experienced 25% less pain and 30% more physical activity than those who weren't.

It has alkaline-forming properties that are necessary for the body. A tablespoon of apple cider vinegar can relieve the pain of heartburn. It has all-around alkalizing properties that the body needs in this age of acid-forming diets.

It is an active ingredient in pineapple and has been shown to reduce bloating and heaviness. It improves blood circulation and prevents blood clots. It also stops menstrual cramps and muscle pain. People with arthritis should use it.

Garlic was the most well-known pain relief in the past. Garlic is used to treat toothache, as well as other skin conditions such acne and psoriasis. Garlic has anti-fungal, anti-inflammatory and pain-relieving properties.

Oats have been shown to reduce menstrual cramps. Oats can also relieve endometriosis. They are rich in magnesium and provide the best source of dietary zinc for women who suffer from painful periods.

A study by Ohio University found that 1 cup of grapes daily reduces back pains and the risk of developing them. Grapes are believed to have nutrients that improve blood circulation and thus relieve pain.

These anti-oxidants kill free radicals which enflame the digestive system, thus reducing the severity of gastrointestinal pain.

There are many practitioners you might already know, in addition to the long list of natural pain relief options. These services may complement one another. Chronic pain can often be a complex and multifaceted issue. It's like an onion that has many layers. It's not unusual to combine several of these services. All of them work together to help remove layers.

The neuromusculoskeletal system is what chiropractors focus on. They also consider the relationship between the spine and the rest of the body. They believe subluxations or misalignment can occur even during birth. Chronic conditions and pain can be created when the body is out of balance. To relieve nerve pressure and promote healing, the chiropractor manipulates the joints. The chiropractor may need to teach the muscles surrounding the spine a "new memory" to ensure pain relief.

Massage therapy is often used in conjunction with other types of physical therapy. Massage therapy focuses on the manipulation of the muscles and connective tissue in the body using a variety techniques. According to the American Heritage dictionary, massage is "the rubbing or kneading parts of the body in order to aid circulation or relax muscles." Chronic pain can often be relieved when muscles are relaxed and capable of functioning as they were intended. There are many types of massage therapy, including deep tissue massages, Swedish massages, Shiatsu, and others.

Chinese medicine is based upon 5000 years worth of tradition. It often includes herbal medicine, acupuncture and massage.

Based on pressure points within the body, stimulates nerves and releases endorphins. Acupuncture inserts needles into the skin along meridians or acupuncture points. Instead of using needles, acupressure uses fingers and other instruments.

It is common to seek physiotherapy for a serious injury or disability. The body usually has limited movement or is unable to perform as intended after an accident. Physiotherapy is a treatment that uses physical techniques to treat the body's injury, disease or deformity. It does not use drugs or surgery. These techniques include stretching, massage, heat treatment, and exercise.

The Canadian Association of Naturopathic Doctors states that "naturopathic medicine" is a unique primary care system that combines modern scientific knowledge with traditional and organic forms of medicine. Naturopathic medicine aims to increase the healing potential of the body and address the root cause of disease. Unfavorable lifestyle choices and poor functioning are indicators of disease. In addition to diet and lifestyle changes, natural therapies including botanical medicine, clinical nutrition, hydrotherapy, homeopathy, naturopathic manipulation and traditional Chinese medicine/acupuncture, may also be used during treatments."

There is a strong connection between essential oils and the olfactory system. There are many herbs that have healing properties and can be used to treat a wide range of chronic conditions. Aromatherapy can be done in many ways. You can light a candle, apply pressure points to your skin, or spritz on a pillow. Basil is used to treat migraines, while lavender is anti-inflammatory.

Hypnotherapy can be described as a skillful verbal communication that helps a client direct their imagination so that they experience desired alterations in sensations and perceptions. It has been proven that hypnotherapy can be used to ease pain during childbirth. Hypnotherapy is self-taught, or can be implemented by a trained therapist.

Simple stretching and yoga are easy practices that can be used in everyday life to relieve stress and maintain good muscle function. You can target specific areas, such as the neck and lower back. These stretches may be taught by a personal trainer or massage therapist. You can practice yoga at home, or with a group of others. There are many types of yoga, from hot yoga to hatha yoga. Yoga focuses on breathing control, meditation and stretching, as well as balance. If you are not comfortable with the practice of yoga, there are other forms.

Chapter 17: Manage Stress and Avoid Stress

Learning a few stress management strategies can help you avoid fatigue. If stress is not managed, it can drain your energy.

If you don't address the issue immediately, extreme stress levels can lead to serious health problems. Stress can cause cognitive dysfunction and affect energy levels, which can have a negative impact on your quality of life. These tips will help you reduce stress and prevent exhaustion.

Be kind to yourself.

Many types of stress can be self-induced. You can eliminate all stress and fatigue by being gentle with yourself. Avoid working too hard until you feel exhausted.

Meditate.

Meditation can be a great way to manage stress. Meditation can help you to improve your cognitive function, increase your energy, and vitality.

You should choose a quiet spot where you won't be disturbed.

When you meditate, be comfortable.

Take deep, slow breaths and close your eyes. Keep your eyes on the breath.

Recognize any distracting thoughts or trivial thoughts that may arise in your mind and bring your attention back to your breathing.

This should take between five and ten minutes.

After a short, silent prayer of thanksgiving, open your eyes.

Regular meditation is essential to reap the benefits. As you improve your meditation practice, you can increase it.

Pray.

Prayers can reduce stress. You will feel more optimistic and have more energy.

Drop perfectionism.

You can set unrealistic standards if you strive for perfection. Perfectionism is one of the best ways to manage stress and anxiety. You must do your best every time. Remember that doing your best is enough.

You have a great sense for humor.

Don't take your life too seriously. You must have a sense of humor if you want to live a happy, stress-free lifestyle. Learn to laugh at yourself. There is always something to smile about, and there are funny things in all situations. You can also find funny videos on YouTube. You will feel instantly good and this will increase your energy.

Talk to someone.

Talking with someone can help you reduce stress and boost your energy. Talking to someone will make you realize that you're not alone in your struggle. It is very therapeutic to talk to someone you trust, care about, and that's what I recommend.

Be clear about your goals.

You can avoid stress and not be too thin by being clear about your goals. Set clear goals for every aspect of your life, including personal development, finances and career.

Prioritize.

You can reduce stress by learning to prioritize tasks. This can help you conserve energy and avoid fatigue. Prioritizing helps you to recognize your body's limits.

Identify what you have control over.

There are certain things you can control and some that you cannot. You can live a happy, stress-free and high-energy life if you focus on what you can control. Learn to let go of what you cannot control, and don't stress about it.

Play.

Most adults don't play anymore. It is important to relax and have fun. Play video games or engage in sports. Spend time with your children if you have them. You will be appreciated by them more.

11. Take deep breaths.

A few deep, slow breaths can help you relax when you feel stressed or tired. Take deep, slow breaths and inhale as far as possible. You will immediately feel the results if you do this for 3-5 times.

You must manage your stress. Anger, jealousy and guilt are all negative emotions that can drain your energy and cause anxiety, depression, and fatigue. Negative emotions can drain your energy and can take away all the positive vibes in your life. These are some ways to manage your emotions.

Forgive yourself.

If you feel guilty for something you did years ago, you will feel overwhelmed and stressed. You can live a happier life by learning to forgive yourself for past mistakes and missteps. Your vitality and health will increase if you can forgive yourself. Your energy levels will rise as a result.

Forgive others.

Grudges can drain your energy and cause anxiety. Learn to forgive people who have wronged you in the past if you want to boost your energy and vitality. It does not mean you condone their actions or that you will accept them back into your life. This is a sign that you are willing to let go and that you want to live the life you deserve.

Create healthy personal boundaries.

Some people are naturally inclined to want to please others. But trying to please everyone at all costs can cause frustration and stress. You can improve your emotions and increase energy by setting healthy boundaries. You can drain your energy by being too friendly to others. Sometimes it is okay to say no to requests that are not in your best interest. This is one of your best ways to avoid stress and fatigue.

You must learn how to manage your emotions if you want to have high levels of energy. Avoid stress wherever possible. It is better to avoid stressful situations if possible.

Chapter 18: More Evidence of Humans as Frugivores

Although the human anatomy has been studied for many centuries, there is still no consensus on what type of diet humans have adapted to. Although it is common to see humans being called "omnivores", this classification comes from the observation of how humans eat under cultural conditions and not what they would eat unconditioned by society.

The lack of clear rules to define what an "omnivore" is, makes it difficult to claim that humans are anatomically "omnivores". An anatomist defines an omnivore to be an animal that is neither an herbivore or a carnivore. An anatomist can't define what something isn't, so omnivores may be considered "non-specialists", meaning they are able to consume both plant and animal matter.

This article presents data that together indicate that humans are strong omnivores. It attempts to use a multidisciplinary approach in categorising human dietary adaptations. A strong frugivore is an animal that eats fruits only or almost entirely and has specialized adaptations to this diet.

This classification, like other frugivorous animals would allow for occasional consumption of animal and insect matter. However, such occasions would be considered special exceptions or contamination rather than regular, deliberate consumption due to biological necessity. An omnivore would eat large amounts of animal matter regularly and would not be considered a strong frugivore.

Classification confusion

Pilbeam (9), describes apes broadly as "herbivores", as opposed to carnivores and omnivores. Yerkes(4) and Yerkes(4) agree that primates should be considered "omnivores". Maier(2) disagrees. There are many opinions on how primates should be classified, including those of chimpanzees and humans. However, there is no consensus. Chivers' research on human digestive system anatomy is not conclusive, but he has done some of the most thorough studies of mammal digestion. In "Diet and Guts"(1), Chivers summarizes that the human gut anatomy is typical of meat-eating or other fast-digestible foods.

His plots however show that the human digestive anatomy is located at the edge and, more importantly, is Cebus capucinus, the white-fronted cauchin. According to The Pictorial Guide To The Living Primates, Cebus capucinus eats 95 types of fruit that make up 65% of its diet, while leaves make up 15%.

The rest of the diet is composed of fruits, nuts, seeds and shoots. Cebus capucinus is frugivore-insectivore, not a carnivore, but they have also been called omnivores. Others have reported that Cebus capucinus makes up to 78% of its diet from fruit, and still call it an omnivore because of its regular consumption of animal foods. Chivers chart shows that C. capucinus may have a digestive system similar to humans.

None of the other omnivore species seem to have an anatomy that is similar to humans, except perhaps the chimpanzee. The chimpanzee is sometimes described as a frugivore or foli-frugivore. However, others refer to it as an omnivore. As we will see, human anatomy differs from that of chimps.

There is currently no system that can reliably classify a species' diet based on its behaviour or anatomy. Anatomical observations may be misleading. Milton(7) points out that while the panda bear's digestive system is similar to that of a carnivore (p. 14), it eats a mostly herbivorous diet. The anatomical traits of all Carnivora species share anatomical traits, which means that they all eat diets that range from pure carnivory through omnivory and frugivory (p. 14).

Chimpanzees prefer a high-fruit diet when there is fruit in season, but they can diversify and include more leaves and meat when there is not enough fruit. Chimpanzees, like humans, have their own food cultures. This means that their diet may not reflect local traditions and habitats. This might seem like an example of an omnivore, but we may accept it as such. However, even rabbits cannibalize their placentas and other "herbivores".

When introduced to animal matter in captivity, herbivorous species may also eat it. Most "herbivores", however, will ingest insect matter and foliage. Wild animals are not able to refuse the chance to eat nutritious food, even if it means that a herbivore is eating its own placenta. This would lead us to conclude that all mammals are "omnivores". However, a general definition does not make a category. Such broad categorisations would allow for similarities to be considered equivalents.

There are obviously issues regarding the quantity, frequency, and type of animal matter that is consumed. These issues need to be clarified before a species is considered an omnivore. This clarification is necessary to distinguish animals that only eat small amounts of flesh or are subject to unusual environmental pressures or domestication from those who eat more regularly and more deliberate. One might argue that omnivores are distinguished from herbivores or carnivores by their ability to change the diet in response to environmental pressures. This behavior is considered evidence of omnivory.

After reading a lot of literature, I can see that academics in this field have not yet produced the same systematic quantified and broadly agreed definitions as those in other scientific disciplines. There are many opinions on the basic dietary characteristics of primates.

Notice: While "animal matter" is usually used to refer to vertebrate flesh in this paper, it may also include insects.

Digestive Anatomy

Humans have a digestive system that is more dominant than that of other primates. The colon is smaller and the intestines are larger. The human digestive system is smaller than that of other primates. Milton(7) states that the human small intestinal tract makes up more than 56% of the total stomach, while the colon only makes up 17 to 23%.

The colon is greater than 45% in all other apes, while the intestines range from 14 to 29% in all others. This confirms Chivers' findings and shows that humans are a distinct species in terms of their digestive anatomy. It is therefore logical to search outside the apes in search of a species that may better match our digestive anatomy. Perhaps monkeys, birds, or bats.

The majority of large primates, including all the great apes, are foli-frugivores. However, they eat some animal matter and the smaller ones are faunivores (Tarsius. sp.). They may also eat fruits (e.g. Galagoides demidoff). Only Callithrix Humeralifer (tasseleared marmoset), and Ateles Paniscus (black spider monkey), eat more that 80% of their diets as fruits (11). The rest comes mainly from leaves or gum, and a small amount from animal matter.

The marmoset with a tassel-eared ear is almost entirely frugivorous. It eats 17% of its diet from gums, which are chemically very similar to fruits. They are primarily a source carbohydrate. Small insects make up 0.5% of the remaining feeding time. Only a few species of 234 primate species are known to exhibit strong frugivory.

An analysis of literature on functional anatomy revealed that leaf is mainly digested in highly sacculated stomachs and haustrated colonies. These adaptations drastically increase the volume of the gut for a given length. This slows down digestion so that bacterial fermentation may occur. Although humans also have haustrated colonies, it is less common than in other apes. Animal matter and fruits are the main foods that digest in the intestines. They can be quickly broken down due to the absence of indigestible cell walls in leaves.

The work of Chivers excludes birds and bats. Only birds and bats are likely to encounter animals that eat only fruits, such as the completely frugivorous pteropodid Bats. Jordano mentions in chapter 'Fruits and Frugivory(5) that strong frugivores also have a gut that is dominated by the intestinales (p.145). According to 16 reports, frugivorous bats like Wahlberg's fruit-bat have small intestines which make up 94% of their total digestive system (16).

spit the fruit fibres out, ingesting only the juices. Jordano points out (p.138), that unlike "omnivores", frugivores don't require any special adaptations or digestive processes to process fruit.

Contrary to Chivers' findings(1), Hladik and Chivers(12) plotted functional mucosa area vs. functional bodies for folivores/faunivores and found that humans fit the frugivore trends. In this study, each trend line was distinct. This method seems to be more accurate than Chivers methods in terms of prediction.

Summary: Digestive anatomy research has shown that the human digestive system is compatible with foods that are more easily digested than those made from tough plant fibres. This ratio of functional body size to surface area is similar to that found in frugivores. Humans fall in the middle of the ratio of colon to intestine for foli-frugivorous animals and the extreme case of juice-eating bats and soft fruit eaters. (see table below). Humans have a dominant digestive system, with the small intestines dominating. This is not only a characteristic shared by frugivores but also to omnivores and other faunivores.

The proportion of Intestine & Colon in Apes and Humans.

Great Ape   Human

Frugivorous Bat

Intestines   14% - 29%   56%   94%

Colon 45%   17% - 23%   4%

Diet   Foli-frugivore   What is the best way to get started?   soft fruit/fruit juices

Fruit   64%*   What is the best way to get started?   100

Fibres 27%*   What is the best way to get started?   ~0 (ejected)

Animal Matter   4%*   What is the best way to get started?   0

* for chimpanzees (The Feeding Ecology Of Apes, Nancy L. Conklin-Brittain,1 Cheryl D. Knott,1 and Richard W. Wrangham)

It is very easy to reduce the complex digestive system to just a few measurements, without considering the chemistry or physiology. The anatomy of the digestive system tends to reflect the food's physical properties, not the source. This makes it difficult to determine the exact details of the diet or could be misleading. However, humans can still be classified as highly frugivorous.

Dental Anatomy

Human dental anatomy is different from that of the great apes. The dominant canine teeth in the great apes are prominent and play an important role in defense, feeding, and display. The rest of the teeth are strikingly similar to human ones. Bonobo and human teeth, for instance, look almost identical as illustrated in the book Bonobo: The

Forgotten Ape(10). This suggests that the diet and dietary strategy are very similar. Contrary to this, the human canine's tooth is not as prominent and has a similar shape and size to the incisors.

This similarity is why human canines are called "incisiform" dogs. It has been suggested(8), that they act as extensions to the incisors, and, by analogy, perform the same function. In herbivores, large and spatulate incisiform canines are common. Pilbeam(8) states that incisors of large size are associated with food procurement tasks. (What must be done to get bite-sized portions, such as eating large fruits with hard skins).

Human dental anatomy is identical to that of frugivorous great-apes. Canine teeth have been added to make it more fruit-based. Canine teeth are still made from a pointed structure, but the evolution of humans must have been so significant that thick enamel outgrowths were preferred.

Digestive Transit

Jordano(5) states that strong frugivores need to eat large amounts of fruits, which they quickly digest and then eliminate. Chivers concludes the human digestive system has been adapted to quickly digested foods(1). Milton's paper(7) argues that the human digestive system remains in its slower-digesting herbivorous ancestral state.

Her digestive transit study was based on modern humans, who are known to be constipated and have many degenerative diseases. Milton's study is based on the assumption that humans are adaptable to eating meat, and Chivers claims meat is fast digested. Why then does Milton's research show subjects only digest slowly as herbivores?

*eg: appendicitis and diverticular diseases, colon cancer, 40% of the UK population are constipated(14), hemorhoids affect approximately a third of people, and 2/3 of the older population.

Milton states that the mean transit time of liquid markers in chimps on high-fiber diets (a more natural situation) is 35.1+–2.3 hours. In humans, it is 38.9–61.6 hours (results with particle markers are similar).

The human doesn't digest cultural "omnivorous", despite having less haustration than a chimp who has to break down hard leaf matter for about a day and half. Burkitts' figures (13), only rural villagers who eat high-fiber diets have transit times comparable with chimpanzees. Contrary to this, people who eat more processed Western foods had transit times of 42.4 hours for UK vegetarians and 83.4-144 hours for naval personnel.

Milton's study found that all the great apes and humans studied had an average of 24 hours between the first appearance of digestive markers. The mean transit time of the archetype "omnivore", a dog, was 37.4 hours. However, this number dropped to 28.7 hours when they ate more fibre (15).

Speedyvet also report mean retention times of around 23 hours for dogs. Both humans and dogs can speed up digestion by increasing their fibre intake and decreasing their meat intake.

The findings of digestive anatomy and research on digestive transit times seem to be in conflict with those on digestion. Domestic dogs are slower to digest meat-based diets than chimpanzees and humans, even though they do so when there is more fibre in their diet. Perhaps mean transit times reflect body size and diet more than anatomy. Research on humans also showed that a reduced transit time (17), which is a risk factor in cancer (17,18). Transit times research seems to be limited to certain species and observations.

Biochemistry

It is not surprising that humans are a departure from great apes in their digestive anatomy. Below is the table showing the nutritional makeup (19) of human breastmilk. It also shows that of great-apes.

Primates	Total Solids (%)	Protein (%)	Fat (%)	Sugar (%)	Ash (%)
* Human	12.5	1.0	4.4	6.9	0.2
Great Apes (*2)	11.5	2.8	3.0	5.5	0.2

The composition of primate milks. (*1) Homo sapiens, Packard, 1982; (*2) Pongo pygmaeus, Pan troglodytes, Ben Shaul, 1962; Gorilla gorilla, Tailor & Tomkinson, 1975;

Milk produced by great apes contains almost three times the amount of protein as human milk and slightly less sugar and fat than human milk. Human babies are born in an immature stage of development. Their large heads must fit through the narrow apertures of the cervix while their bodies are still developing. Given the infant's lack of development and relative immobility, we can assume that human infants require significantly less protein than other apes.

Desomatisation is the characteristic lack of human head development compared to the body is known. It is a trait that is common in primates, as Terrance Dacon explains in his book The Symbolic Species' (20). Harper's Biochemistry 24th Ed. states that the average male body contains 17% protein (p.6), most of it muscle. While muscle contains 18 to 20% of the protein in human body, brain tissue has only 8% protein (21), and twice as much fat. Brain tissue also has a longer life span than muscles, which is why the proteins are so much more durable. Therefore, brain tissue has a lower protein requirement than muscles.

Based on Nancy Lou Conklin Brittain's research, these figures are approximate. 22), shows that wild fruits are a good source of protein and carbohydrate for chimpanzees. It is clear that chimpanzees are able to eat fruits in large amounts, as their adult nutritional requirements are less than those needed for growth and development.

A similar situation should be expected for humans. They have a lower protein intake and a higher need for sugars to fuel their brains. Since glucose is the primary metabolite in brain tissue, this analogy can be used. Omnivores like the dog require far more animal protein to develop and grow normally.

As one would expect from a species that eats a lot of fruits, the human biochemistry is not able to handle high levels of protein. Infant birth weight is affected by a high dietary protein intake (between 100 and 150 grams per day). A deadly condition known as 'rabbit starvation' can be induced by higher protein intake (24). However, the figures range from 35% to 50% of daily calories(24), 23.

Similar conditions have not been observed in unequivable or faunivores. Dogs that are fed grains-based pet foods are known to have skin and hair problems. Humans are not affected by these conditions.

Many anthropologists love the theory that animal matter has provided humans with enough calories per unit of food over their plant-based diet to enable them to develop larger brains. Deacon (20) points out that humans do not grow larger heads, but smaller bodies.

This energy boost from high-calorie foods may be part of a maternal diet strategy(2).

Speth (23), however, suggests that during this time women often experience an aversion to meat and odours of meat, while cravings for carbohydrate foods are most common. Speth speculates that pregnant women may consume too much meat.

Humans also lack the ability to synthesize vitamin C. This is a characteristic that is only found in herbivores such as great apes. These and other fundamental differences in anatomy, physiology, and behavior should prevent humans from being placed with other omnivores. They also support the theory that humans are strong fumigvores.

Acid reflux is a condition in which a person ingests large amounts of animal products and then eats low-protein meals. In anticipation of animal protein, the stomach will produce a certain amount of acid every day. This buffer is very powerful.

The production of sulphuric acids in the colon is another danger of eating high-sulphurous foods, such as meat or other sulphurous substances. The gut bacteria will convert the undigested sulphur amino acid into hydrogen sulphide. This combines with water to make sulphuric acids. According to New Scientist (26), this is believed to promote many diseases. The human colon seems to be better adapted for plant food than meat.

Behaviour

The Yerkes spent a lot of their lives studying primates literature and working with them. Tuttle(4) states that Yerkes(4) and Yerkes eschewed using the term "facile", as they believed most apes (especially infants) would easily eat a wide variety of human foods.

It is likely that this is the same situation where we find humans with no strong instincts to eat certain foods in their natural state. Some of the drives that are genuinely present in humans and therefore 'instincts' are the sweet tooth, the repulsion to bitter substances, and the 'Pica" phenomenon. The bitter leaves and tasteless fruits that chimpanzees consume are not something humans would eat.

A strong instinctive attraction to prey species' smell is not something we see in humans. The fruit-eating species can locate their food visually. Architypical "omnivores", such as bears and pigs, have acute senses of smell and can find buried food. Visual tracking of prey is an effective way to obtain some types of insects.

According to Chivers(3), humans can only be omnivores if they use food processing technologies (p. 4), which allow them to make tough animal and plant matter edible. He goes on to say that Omnivorism is impossible because any digestive system cannot handle large amounts of plant matter, fruit, and animal matter.

What would ancient human ancestors eat if they didn't have fire or hunting tools? Many paleoanthropology books suggest that humans were frugivorous. However, there are often suggestions that animals were eaten as part of their diets, as either scavenged carcasses, or as insect matter.

Regardless of the truth, modern humans don't like the smells of dead animals. Humans do not eat animals in their raw form or in the condition of decay that animal food is found in nature. While one might think this is due to cultural conditioning, the fact remains that raw animal matter can pose a host of problems, including parasites and toxic substances found in necrotic tissue.

This may be why humans make so much effort to mask the true flavour and appearance of animal foods using herbs and other, often plant-derived seasonings. It is hardly fitting for any carnivore and omnivore. All humans, however, are attracted to the sweet smells and flavours of fruits and vegetables.

How many people would choose to eat the more nutritious animal matter if they were given the option of a live rabbit, cow or chicken? If humans were given the freedom to choose, but are deprived of food processing technology, they will resort to eating frugivory.

Confounding Questions

Milton(7) stated in a 1904 publication that the physiologists Elliot-Smith and Barclay Smith had said that the human stomach was more like that of an herbivore than an Omnivore. These conclusions were either ignored or forgotten or people believed them to be incorrect. The next century saw far more comparative biology, but despite or because of thousands of dissections research has not come to an agreement on what man's naturalistic diet is.

Comparative biologists face many axiomatic problems that make it difficult to produce usefully precise results. The less one can find a species similar enough to man, the further one travels in the genetic gap between the subject and the animal being compared.

Many anthropologists have made the chimpanzee a focal point of their research. However, an examination of its teeth and faeces, as well as a tasting of the food it eats should convince us that we don’t share a common diet. Chimpanzees have a very different evolutionary history than humans, and are not related to any human ancestors. Chimpanzees, in any event, have their own food cultures as well as environmental challenges that can confuse analysis.

Because of the huge gap between great apes, others have decided to concentrate on man's recent ancestors. They can either examine fossil finds or look at modern hunter-gatherers. Lewin (25) stated that fossils cannot be used to determine if they are our ancestors or just our cousins.

Each new fossil discovery is added to the evolutionary tree. This makes the tree more complicated and requires that the linear view of our supposed ancestry, which is the only one presented, be modified. Lewontin states that most fossils of different ages can't be linked in a linear order, but are a small selection from many parallel lines.

Enculturation can be a confusing influence even in chimpanzees, so what chance do we have of finding a naturalistic diet for ancient hominids. Even if we could, how do we convince people that their diets are healthy?

Similar questions apply to contemporary hunter-gatherers. Are they really healthy? There are certainly lessons to be learned, but there is a lot of empirical nutrition research that is often overlooked in the hopes of discovering a dietary optimal in cavemen and apes.

It is crucial to have a set of rigidly defined and mutually exclusive categories, as well as a method for establishing a dietary taxonomy before you can embark on your mission. Inadequate systems have led to confusion and free-for-all naming.

Bibliography

Jones/Martin/Pilbeam, The Cambridge Encyclopedia of Human Evolution,

Cambridge University Press 1992

Chivers et al., Food Acquisition And Processing in Primates, N.Y. Plenum Press, 1984

Chivers and colleagues, The Digestive Systems in Mammals: Food Form And Function, Cambridge University Press 1994

Tuttle R. H. Apes of the World Communication, Mentality, and Ecology. William Andrew Publishing, 1986

Jordano P., 'Fruits and Frugivory', in Seeds: The Ecology of Regeneration in Plant Communities, 2nd Edition, Fenner et al., CAB International Publishing, 2000

Whiten A., Cultures in Chimpanzees, Nature, 399, 682-685, 1999

Milton K., 'A Hypothesis To Explain the Role Of Meat-Eating In Human Evolution', Evolutionary Anthropology Vol. 8:11-21

Pilbeam D., 'Human Evolution' course Harvard College, Science B-27 handouts, Section 3 - Anatomy II: The Cranium, Mandible And Dentition

Pilbeam D., Science B-27 handouts, Spring 2001: Chapter 4--Human-chimp contrasts

De Waal F. Lanting F. Bonobo: Bonobo, Uni. Calif. Press 1997

Rowe N. The Pictorial Guide To Living Primates, Pogonias Press N.Y. 1996

Hladik C. and coauthors, "Diet, Gut Size and Brain Size", Current Anthropology vol. 40, no. 40, no.

Burkitt D. and coauthors, "Effects of dietary fiber on stools, transit times and their role in the causation and prevention of disease," The Lancet, 30 December 1972.

NACNE, "Proposals for nutritional guidance for health education in Britain", The Health Education Council Sep. 1983

Burrows, CF and colleagues, "Effects fiber on digestibility, transit time in dogs", J Nutr, 1982 Sep. 112(9):1726-32.

Makanya A. and coauthors, "Gut Morpology and Morpometry in the Epauletted Wahlberg's Fruit Bat", Acta Biol Hung 2001,52(1):75-89

Hughes R. Hughes R,.

Silvester K. and colleagues, "Effects of meat and resistant starch in fecal excretion apparent N-nitroso compounds or ammonia from large bowel of the human being" Nutr Cancer 1997;29(1), 13-23

Juan T. Borda and Exequiel Patino, "The Composition and Importance of Primates' Milk in Selecting Formulas For Hand-Rearing", Laboratory Primate Newsletter, vol. 36 no. 36 no. 2, Apr.

Deacon T. (1997), The Symbolic Species Penguin Books, pp. 165-174

McIlwain H., and Bachelard H.S. Biochemistry and the Central Nervous System. Edinburgh: Churchill Livingstone 1985

Conklin-Brittain N. et al., 'Relating Chimpanzee Diets to Potential Australopithecus Diets',

Speth J., "Protein selection strategies and avoidance strategies", in Philosophical Transactions of the Royal Society of London, vol. 334, no. 334, no.

Douglas F., "Cut the Carbs", New Scientist, 18 Mar 2000, no.2230

R. Lewontin. 'It Ain't Necessarily so'. Granta 2000.

Gail Vines, 'A Gut Feeling', New Scientist, vol 159 issue 2146 - 08 August 1998, page 26

Hydrogen sulphide is a bacterial toxin that can cause ulcerative colitis. Max Pitcher and John Cummings, Gut, vol. 39, p1 (1996)

Glenn Gibson, Sandra Macfarlane, and George Macfarlane, FEMS Microbiology Ecology vol 12, p.117 (1993). Metabolic interactions in the human large intestinale involving methanogenic and sulphate-reducing bacteria

William Roediger and colleagues, Gastroenterology vol. 104, p. 802 (1993).

The large intestine in nutrition and disease by John Cummings, Institute Danone, ISBN 2930151021, http://www.danone-institute.com (1997)

Chapter 19: Your Lifestyle

"Men worry more about what's not visible than what they can see."

~ Julius Caesar

We worry every day. It seems like this is a natural human trait to prepare for every situation. It's almost an instinctive animal instinct to protect oneself. Because of how 21st-century life is lived, however, we often do the opposite. We don't eat healthy meals and eat too fast as we don't have the time. We are our worst enemies because we don't get enough sleep. We drink, smoke, and use vapor substitutes for cigarettes. Most of us rush through our lives so fast that we are guilty of neglecting others that, if done to them, would be considered cruelty. Let's take a look at areas you can improve on to reduce stress.

The digestive system

This can lead to physical pain if you don't properly eat. If your food isn't properly processed, you can feel heartburn and unwell. This is an area that you should work on if you've ever eaten a sandwich in a rush because you don’t have the time to chew it properly. When you abuse your body to such an extent, eventually it complains and eventually causes you stress. It can't handle what you do to it. You're not properly eating your food and are likely to be swallowing air. Are you suffering from wind? Are you feeling short of breath? Do you feel panicked? Are you feeling pains in your chest or stomach?

It is important to take care of your digestive system. Anxiety can lead to binging, which is when people overeat and neglect their digestive system. What does all this have to do anxiety and depression? You might not realize it, but there is more to it. You don't feel good if you have low self-esteem and then cause your body pain. The pain can make you feel like you're dying. This kind of treatment can only be tolerated by the body before it begins to complain. It is important to eat healthy foods, sit down and enjoy them.

Also, you need to reduce the amount of fast food that you consume and focus on providing your body with a balanced diet. This will ensure that your body can function properly. This means that you need to be aware of the negative effects your diet has on your body. Pay attention to labels. Avoid colorings and foods high in calories. You will feel much better and your body will be grateful. You may feel stressed by certain foods. This is something you should know if you've ever had to do. Be aware of what you eat and how it was prepared.

Your sleep

Stress freaks have told me that they are able to not sleep well and I believe that this will eventually happen for physiological reasons. Your body was designed to require all natural human activities in order to stay healthy. You will soon find yourself a lot less smart than your body if you cut out one of these activities. Then, the inevitable suffering you'll face will follow. Sleep deprivation is a major factor in anxiety and depression. There's a good reason. Your body is constantly replenishing itself, even though you may not realize it. There are many stages to sleep and each stage leads to another in a specific order. You can't let your body heal itself if you don’t get REM sleep. When you're actually asleep, REM sleep means that your subconscious can solve all of your problems. You can also burn calories and heal injuries like muscle fatigue while you sleep. You don't get all the benefits if you refuse to go to bed or have a short sleep. In the daytime, it is quite normal to feel anxious, stressed, and panicked more often than someone who goes to bed every 8-9 hours.

You are actually fighting your body instead of allowing it to do its work. Imagine running a car 24x7 and not caring about it. This is the equivalent to what people do to their bodies when they aren't sleeping. You are ready for the next day when you get enough sleep. You may feel lethargic if you don't get enough sleep. It can also cause you to be weaker and reduce your ability to concentrate.

Cigarettes and drinks

Stimulants are a favorite of all and we thrive on them. All stimulants, including coffee, tea, and cold beverages, can increase the body's stress levels. You would expect positive results if you took a handful of caffeine tablets. Your body will respond differently if you take them in small amounts. If you push it too far, your nervous system kicks in and says, "I cannot cope with this." This causes anxiety and stress. One patient was proud that she quit coffee, but she switched to energy drinks with equal amounts of caffeine. She also smoked two packs per day of cigarettes. This is all a habitual, but it affects the way you breathe and how you hyperventilate.

Your adrenaline levels can get too high and you feel anxious. Stress, anxiety, and worry are the only ways your body can get rid of this excess nervous energy. You are your worst enemy. But before you start cursing yourself, take a look at your life and try to balance it. You can have everything in moderation at work. It doesn't mean you have to give up on the things you love, but it is important to do so:

*A varied and healthy diet is important

*Include plenty of fruits and vegetables

Drink lots of water

*Sleep at Night

*Sit down, and properly chew your food

*Exercise regularly

All of these are lifestyle choices. We gave you an example of a man who worries more about what he can't see, than about what he can see. This is true in all aspects of life, and also applies to people's lifestyles. It's the things that people worry about.

*Not being capable of swallowing

*It is difficult to breathe

*Getting into a panic situation

These may be feelings you've experienced in the past, but they are over now if you make lifestyle changes. We will discuss the reasons you feel these feelings and the first steps you can take to overcome them. But, lifestyle changes are essential. Reduce stress-related behaviors.

This book doesn't mean you have to throw it away. It just asks you to give up something that you don't want to give up. You just need to take responsibility and stop smoking, quit drinking soda, and replace your excess coffee with another type of coffee. It doesn't mean you have to give up on the things you love. Be aware of these things and find good things to balance them.

You panic because your balance is out of whack. You aren't treating your body properly. You are more likely to get your life out of control, and you're more susceptible to physical illness, anxiety, and other issues. If you take this chapter in a positive light, you can lower your odds of getting into trouble and allow yourself to move on to the next chapters knowing that you've done something to get your body back under control. You will feel more powerful when you do this. You will feel more confident in your ability to lose weight or cope with any difficulties. You'll be able to breathe more easily. Your body will heal itself and you'll be able to sleep better. You will eat at the correct pace and not feel deprived because of your digestive problems.

You can improve your lifestyle and reduce stress by being conscious of what you control. Good health is dependent on the routine of your daily life. Your body will be at its best when you get enough sleep. You will experience better health and the healing process of sleep can take place. You will eat foods that make you feel good, not comfort food. And you will become more aware of the things you need in your life to make it less stressful, especially if mindfulness is your guide.

Your mind can rest when it is free from stress. This makes problem solving much more easy. Your subconscious is able kick in and assist you with any problems you have. If you overload your mind with negativity, it will stop working for you.

Many people don't know that they are their worst enemies. The world sees a person's mind and how they interact. Positive thoughts and healthy thinking will lead you to positive emotions. Negative vibes are easy to pick up and people will likely send them back. Your attitude to life matters. You can only expect chaos if you approach life in a hurry. You will find more peace of mind if you approach it with kindness and positivity.

I can remember trying to change my diet. I discovered that I was eating boring food and instead of trying new foods, I tried Woks and created many delicious options. I loved eating pineapples. It was easy to see that adding color to your diet is a way to make it healthier. I began to use bell peppers more often than I did before and I really enjoyed the new combinations that I was able to make. It doesn't mean you have to eat boring food. In fact, your food can be as boring as what you make. You will find out how new foods can enhance your meals, and that you enjoy sharing them with friends and family. It is possible that you may be influencing their lives in a positive way.

Stress levels are directly related to your lifestyle. Take a look at your daily life and determine what an average day looks like. Ask yourself these questions:

*How many hours of exercise can I do in 24 hours?

*How much water should I drink?

*How much exercise should I do?

*How many quality hours of sleep can I get?

Your lifestyle and interactions with others are the key to reducing stress levels.

Chapter 20: Compassion Fatigue

Care givers can experience this type of fatigue. Care givers are often affected by compassion fatigue. They experience normal symptoms of chronic stress due to the caregiving work they do every day. The caregiving sector is a popular career choice for people who are already suffering from compassion fatigue. This is due to the fact that people are used to living with traumatized, helpless and suffering animals. Compassion fatigue can be treated by addressing past traumas and pain so that you can live a happier, healthier lifestyle. Regular exercise is important for your physical and mental health. The healing process is enhanced by healthy eating habits, regular exercise, social activities, journaling, and restful sleep. You can achieve full recovery faster if you have the right mindset and are able to integrate your work into daily life.

These measures can help you avoid fatigue:

Healthy, balanced meals that meet all your nutritional needs are key to a healthy body. Supplements are not recommended to supply essential nutrients to the body. Get at least 8 glasses water each day. Reduce the amount of processed, sugary, fatty and deep-fried foods you eat.

You should eat throughout the day. Short breaks are allowed for snacks. Regularly scheduled meals regulate energy supply. Do not skip meals.

You should have a regular and appropriate sleeping schedule. To promote uninterrupted sleep, make your bedroom more comfortable. However, sleeping pills are not recommended for use to induce sleep. You should instead seek the advice of your doctor.

Every day, exercise. Small exercises, such as using stairs instead of lifts, can be incorporated into your workday. Regular exercise can reduce fatigue and improve your sleep quality.

Regular medical checks are important. You will be able to identify any conditions that could cause fatigue and have them addressed immediately. You can identify any stressors and make changes to your life in order to avoid them. Don't wait until you feel depressed before seeking help from professionals. You can organize your work and break down difficult tasks into smaller pieces so that you can focus on the important things without putting too much pressure on your body. Maintain regular breaks between tasks.

Chapter 21: Extra Tips To Help Out

You can still find many ways to combat chronic fatigue and feel better quickly. These are simple changes that you can make to your day. Sometimes it's just a new outlook. These tips will help you get to where you need to go to beat fatigue and make your day more enjoyable and less stressful.

Tip #1: Avoid overexertion

You don't want to have a relapse, or worsen your chronic fatigue. So you should try to avoid overexerting yourself to the best of you. You shouldn't push yourself too hard, even if you feel well. If you do this, you will relapse and feel worse again. There is a medical condition you must be aware of in order to not push yourself beyond your limits and put too much pressure on yourself.

Tip #2: Keep Stress Away

You can do it however you like. If you want to combat chronic fatigue and avoid a relapse, you will need to stop doing this. Chronic fatigue can make you feel tired and deplete your energy. You can try many relaxation techniques until you find one that helps you keep stress at bay.

Tip #3 Keep a Journal

Keep a journal to track all triggers. You can have chronic fatigue from activities or people that are emotionally draining. It can be difficult to identify your triggers, but if you take the time to write them down, you will be able to avoid them. It's important to know the causes of stress, how much sleep you get, and what daily activities might be contributing to it.

Tip #4: Exercise Enough, but Not Too Much

While you can't completely avoid exercising, you should make sure you don't overexert yourself if you have chronic fatigue. Exercise is essential for your health. However, you don't have to do too much if you are experiencing fatigue. While most people can handle an hour or 30 minutes of exercise, someone with chronic fatigue might only be capable of doing fifteen minutes at a stretch. You can keep track of times when exercise is too hard if you already keep a journal.

Tip #5 Stay Hydrated

Water can make a big difference. Water can make all the difference in having energy or not. You will feel drained and unable to do any tasks without feeling even more tired. Drinking enough water will increase your energy and alertness, as well as improve concentration.

Tip #6 Keep a healthy weight

Although there are many ways to combat fatigue, you will feel more fatigue if your weight is too low. If you want to reduce fatigue symptoms, try to maintain a healthy weight. If you are following a diet that reduces fatigue, you should also ensure that you maintain a healthy weight.

Keep this in mind:

Chronic fatigue is a difficult battle that can lead to unresolved problems. You should try to find a way to reduce stress and anxiety if you have chronic fatigue. You can find natural remedies and herbal treatments to help you manage your fatigue. It is important to not give up on chronic fatigue. You need to be able to find the right balance between your work schedule and how you handle it.

Chapter 22: Understanding the Stress Response

Long Term Exposure Impairs Health

Chronic Stress

Stress can manifest in many ways, both psychologically and environmentally. The former can be the fear of losing his job, while the latter refers to the need to complete work by a given deadline. These stress situations can cause physiological changes like a quickening or pounding heartbeat. Occasionally, muscles may tighten and one will start to sweat.

The fight-or flight response is collectively known as stress reactions (Wikipedia Contributors 2019, 2019). This survival mechanism allows people and all mammals to quickly respond to life-threatening situations. A well-planned sequence of events is put into action almost immediately. The sequence includes a variety of physiological and hormonal responses that help to confront and overcome the threat. Sometimes, the body reacts too strongly to simple situations like traffic jams and family problems.

Researchers have discovered the reasons and mechanisms behind these reactions through careful research. Researchers also discovered the negative effects of prolonged stress on physical and psychological health. The body can be affected by repeated stress activation. Research shows that chronic stress can cause brain changes, increase blood pressure, and clog arteries. These changes can lead to depression, anxiety, or addiction. Some evidence suggests that obesity could be caused by direct mechanisms, such as eating more or indirectly through reduced exercise and sleep.

The Brain's Response to Stress

The brain is the first to trigger stress alarms. It does this in the same way that one experiences the oncoming car. The amygdala receives information from the eyes and ears, and processes the emotions. The amygdala interprets the images and sounds and sends distress signals to the hypothalamus if there's danger.

Stress Responses

Stress can activate many brain regions. The Amygdala acts as an emotion-processing center, while the hypothalamus is a command center (Pessoa 2010, 2010). The autonomic nervous systems activates the fight or flight response and the hypothalamus is responsible for communicating with it. The functions of the autonomic nervous systems include heartbeat, breathing and dilation and constriction blood vessels. It has two parts, the parasympathetic and sympathetic nervous systems.

Parasympathetic nervous systems triggers the first fight-or flight response. It is similar to a car's gas pedal. Instantly, the body experiences a surge of energy which allows it to quickly respond to dangers. Parasympathetic nervous systems act as a brake, helping the person to relax. After danger passes, it calms the body.

The Sympathetic Nervous System's Action

The autonomous nerves are activated, and the signal from amygdala reaches adrenal glands via the sympathetic nervous system. The glands respond immediately by pumping the epinephrine hormonal hormone. This hormone is also known as the adrenaline, which enters the bloodstream. This causes the heartbeat to beat faster and the bloodstream to circulate epinephrine. Staughton (2019), states that the hypothalamus will signal the adrenal glands (adrenaline), to release epinephrine into the bloodstream. Then you're off to the races...or the battleground!" Other physiological changes include an increase in pulse rate and rising bloodpressure. The blood flow to all vital organs, including the heart and muscles, has increased. This will result in a rise in breath rate, which will cause the airways to become larger. This is done to increase oxygen intake. This increases alertness by pushing more oxygen to the brain. The stimulation of all senses results in sharper sight and hearing. Epinephrine can also increase blood sugar and fat levels by removing them from temporary storage. These nutrients are absorbed into the bloodstream and give rise to increased energy.

These changes take very little time, so the person does not know what is happening. Although the brain's visual center processes these changes normally, the change happens quickly due to the efficient wiring between the amygdala and hypothalamus. This is how people leap out of cars' way without thinking about why.

Follow up action

The hypothalamus activates the second component of the stress response system after the initial epinephrine spike. This happens through the HPA-axis which consists of the hypothalamus and adrenal glands as well as the pituitary and pituitary.

The sympathetic nervous system communicates with the HPA by sending hormone signals to keep the pedal down. If there is a continuous presence of danger, the hypothalamus secretes corticotropin-releasing hormone (CRH) that goes to the pituitary gland and triggers the release of adrenocorticotropic hormone (ACTH). Alschuler (2016). "ACTH binds with receptors on adrenal cortex and stimulates adrenal production of cortisol." ACTH travels up to the adrenal glands, activating cortisol release. The level of cortisol starts to decrease once the threat is over. The parasympathetic nervous systems, which regulates stress, acts as a brake and reduces cortisol levels.

Conclusion

We are grateful that you downloaded this book.

I hope you found this book helpful in understanding the essential aspects of Chronic Fatigue Syndrome.

CFS is still not fully understood. It is still a serious problem. Patients, advocates, and experts are all working together to improve the understanding of this condition. Although there is no proven treatment, it is better to follow the methods described here than not doing anything about the condition.

Next, consult your doctor about how to approach CFS. This applies to you as well as your loved ones. Find out how others are dealing with this condition by looking for other people.

We are grateful and wish you all the best!

www.ingramcontent.com/pod-product-compliance
Lightning Source LLC
Chambersburg PA
CBHW071840080526
44589CB00012B/1072
9781774851678